The First Pregnancy
An Integrating Principle in Female Psychology

Research in Clinical Psychology, No. 13

Peter E. Nathan, Series Editor

Henry and Anna Starr Professor of Psychology
Chairman, Department of Clinical Psychology
Rutgers, the State University of New Jersey

Other Titles in This Series

The First Pregnancy
An Integrating Principle in Female Psychology

by
Jellemieke C. Hees-Stauthamer
Clinical Psychologist
Academic Medical Center
Utrecht, Netherlands

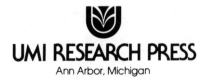

UMI RESEARCH PRESS
Ann Arbor, Michigan

Produced and distributed by
UMI Research Press
an imprint of
University Microfilms International
A Xerox Information Resources Company
Ann Arbor, Michigan 48106

Library of Congress Cataloging in Publication Data

Hees-Stauthamer, Jellemieke C. (Jellemieke Christine), 1950-
  The first pregnancy.

  (Research in clinical psychology ; no. 13)
  "Revision of the author's dissertation, Wright
Institute, 1982"—Verso t.p.
  Bibliography: p.
  Includes index.
  1. Pregnancy—Psychological aspects. 2. Children,
First-born. 3. Pregnant women—Attitudes. I. Title.
II. Series.
RG560.H44   1985   618.2'001'9   85-5791
ISBN 0-8357-1657-0 (alk. paper)

Often, as I wrote this work, I wondered, "What were my mother's thoughts as she held my twin and me in her womb? Did she ever anticipate the things which have come to pass since that time—and today, when I dedicate this work to her?"

In the privacy of personal experience every woman pregnant for the first time struggles for meaning, comes to terms with her fate or fails to do so, just as her ancestors have done for untold generations.

—Marie Jahoda
November 1973

Contents

Preface

This book is based on a study I conducted a few years ago, which grew out of my clinical work with children and their parents. When I see a child in therapy, it is my practice to ask the parents for a careful and detailed developmental history of their child. I ask the parents to begin at the beginning—when the idea of having a child together first came up between them—and to proceed from there through conception, pregnancy, labor, and delivery, on up to the present time when they bring their child to me.

There is much to be learned from this kind of history taking. It allows me to see the relationship of the parents at work as they help or hinder each other in recalling the events surrounding the integration of their child into their relationship. Equally important, it allows the parents to rediscover the richness and complexity of their child's history and to remember their earlier struggles and efforts on the child's behalf. Finally, it also helps establish that therapy is a collaborative enterprise which may well call for accommodations in the family system as the work with the child unfolds.

It was in the course of doing this work and taking such histories that I was time and time again struck by the frequent links between the dynamics of events occurring during the child's prenatal history and the dynamics of the presenting problem for which the parents were seeking help. The complex of feelings surrounding the circumstances of conception, the course of pregnancy, and the events of labor, delivery, and the early weeks of life often seemed to "set the stage" for subsequent events between the parents and/or between the parents and the child.

One mother, for example, whom I shall call Mrs. J., consulted me about her 15-year-old daughter. She told the following story. She had two daughters but was having particular difficulty with the younger. She was concerned about the "vagueness" and difficulty of her relationship with this child, her daughter's conflict and disinterest with school work, and her tendency to stay away from home without permission. When I asked for a history, it appeared that she had conceived her daughter at an awkward time. Sensing that her marriage was faltering and that she might need to provide for herself in the future, Mrs. J. had just started a course of demanding professional studies when she learned she was pregnant. She decided both to have the child and to stay in school, despite the difficulties involved. Her pregnancy was very stressful. She had constant nausea and gained only 10 pounds throughout the nine months. After her daughter's birth, she stayed married and finished her studies. When her youngest was 10, however, she ended the marriage. She left both daughters with her husband while she went to an urban area to look for work. Later, she reclaimed her daughters and brought them to live with her.

When I talked with her daughter, she spoke about her anger at her mother for abandoning her when she went to look for work. She resented having been left with her father, whom she did not like, and suspected that her mother was not really connected to her. The structural elements of this situation—vagueness of emotional connection between mother and child, discontent in the child-mother-father relationship, conflict over work and staying away from home—replicate the emotional constellation of events during Mrs. J.'s pregnancy.

There are many vicissitudes in any child's development, and such links between prenatal and postnatal aspects of a child's connection with the family are not always so clear. Nevertheless, their occurrence was frequent enough so that I began to pay particular attention to pregnancy as a period from which much could be learned about the earliest aspects of a mother's connection with her child.

From the clinical material, it seemed that attention to the expectant mother was central to tracing the antecedents of the child's relationship to the family and the outside world. Her experience of gestation and parturition, her fantasies and feelings during this period appeared to play a crucial part in determining her attitude toward the child and the quality of their unfolding relationship. The objective "reality" of this time seemed intricately bound up with the woman's subjective sense of her situation and her assessment of her partner. In this respect, one pregnancy could differ sharply from another. Mrs. J.'s experience of her first pregnancy, for example, was quite different from her second. Her first pregnancy went smoothly, she had no physical symptoms, and she looked forward to becoming a mother in the context of a more secure marital relation. Her relationship with her first daughter was generally harmonious, characterized by an ease of interaction sorely lacking in her relationship with her younger child.

The more I became interested in the experience of pregnancy as a dynamic component in the formation of mother-infant and family relations, the more complex and intriguing the questions became. Often first or subsequent pregnancies seemed tied to marital difficulties. Input from the expectant mother's relatives, friends, colleagues, and her doctor also had their effect. Again and again, the main thing, however, seemed to be how the confluence of these factors affected the woman's sense of herself. Her hopes and fears for herself and her child, her sense of being changed by the child as well as molding the child from within, all led to a gradual definition of herself as mother or, more specifically, as mother to this particular child.

Finally, I decided to pursue my questions in a more formal way. So began this study of four women, over 30 and pregnant for the first time. Given the increasing number of women today who are attempting to integrate professional concerns with motherhood, I decided to study four highly educated women. I felt their experience of pregnancy, in the context of different levels of professional commitment and different levels of development in their careers, would yield some interesting insights into the interplay between "love and work" in these women's lives.

Acknowledgments

Gratitude is perhaps too mean a word to encompass my feelings as I reflect on the unfailing help received from many quarters while working on this book.

First and foremost I would like to express my deep appreciation to the women who participated in this study. They gave unstintingly of their time and of themselves during a very special period of their lives. I feel privileged to have shared it with them and remain grateful for the openness with which they invited me into their private world.

Dr. Mervin Freedman of San Francisco State University has my special gratitude for his faith, steadfast patience, and critical guidance: without which this book might never have been undertaken, much less completed. Dr. Ben Tong of the Wright Institute, Berkeley, deserves hearty thanks for his belief in the merits of qualitative research and his valuable criticism at all stages of this work. I am further indebted to Dr. Hugh Clegg, child psychologist, whose own sensitive work with children and their parents remains a source of inspiration, and who often managed to revitalize me during dark hours along the way.

Recognition is also due to Joan Roemer and Ginny Irvine, whose help and consultation contributed greatly to the collection of data for this project.

Dr. Jack Engler of Harvard University and Dr. Charles Hampden-Turner of the Wright Institute, Berkeley, are thanked for their careful critique of the manuscript in its earlier form, while I remain grateful to Helen Harvey for her editorial expertise and standard of excellence which proved invaluable at later stages.

Warm thanks go to Dr. Erika Fromm of the University of Chicago for sharing with me her own experience of pregnancy as well as my sense that childbearing offers something of particular value in a woman's life. Her professional support, and especially her personal friendship, greatly enhanced my pleasure in writing about this topic.

I wish to extend special thanks to Cephas Stauthamer and Hidde de Vries: Cephas for teaching me about the art of life and stimulating my creative efforts, and Hidde for his deep personal interest in seeing this work accomplished. Both of them supported me with their shared anticipations as did friends Leon Finney, Karen Shatzkin, Barbara Mercer, Peter Ryan, Gerda Cooper-Rasker, and Dominique Sénegas. Their warmth and encouragement were invariably a source of refreshment and renewal.

Every undertaking needs a personal muse to feed the spirit when it runs dry. My own muse was Richard Hees, whose courage and tenderness even led to a new beginning once this work was done.

Since finishing this book I have been fortunate enough to have a first pregnancy and child of my own. Reviewing the assumptions and results presented in this work from the standpoint of personal experience, I am left even more convinced of pregnancy's emotional significance as an integrating principle in female psychology. In this context I wish to express my heartfelt gratitude to my daughter, Hiske Leona.

Finally, for their generous financial assistance I want to thank the Danforth Foundation.

Introduction

I've become more quiet, more inward . . . I also feel less competitive and more competent.

I feel very alone about pregnancy. People give me a lot of advice, but don't listen.

I am experiencing a major reorientation in my life. My life with my husband, my own goals and aspirations will be drastically affected by this tiny being.

The theme of my pregnancy, the alone thing, became focused. It was that I am alone and no one can do anything to alter that. I got through that aloneness and realized that nothing from the outside can make me whole. I am whole.

The four women in the present study who voiced these feelings reacted to pregnancy in different ways, but all agreed that becoming a mother profoundly changed their lives. The role of pregnancy and the psychological phenomena involved in their journey from being women without children to being mothers is the object of this study.

The birth of a first child is a time of significant transition for a woman and the network of relationships which comprise her world. Simultaneous physiological, psychological, and social changes surround this event and make it one with far-reaching consequences, for with the arrival of the child a "family" is also born. The dyadic couple becomes a triadic, nuclear unit, transformed from individuals without children to "parents." At the same time, the emotional demands and daily realities of infant care may present unforeseen challenges to the structuring of occupational and sexual roles envisaged by the parents prior to the birth. How these challenges are met varies, depending on a number of interpersonal, sociocultural, and ideological factors, but their resolution often leads to accommodations which profoundly influence a woman's life.

In taking up pregnancy as an aspect of feminine psychological development, this study adventures into an area generally neglected. The notion that pregnancy is a period of psychological as well as physiological gestation is comparatively recent, although the suspicion that becoming a mother changes something about a woman is reflected in earliest mythology. Exactly how pregnancy is an integral part of this transformation is still not well understood. By studying a small number of pregnancies in detail, this study attempts to derive in-depth psychological information from the direct analysis of subjective experience. The pregnant woman's sense of self, her experience of changes occurring in her body, and her partner's and her reaction to the conception and gestation are examined at both imaginative, fantasy levels and realistic, "cognitive" levels.

The present study views conception, and the events in life which lead up to it, as the cardinal point from which to consider the psychology of the individual. The infant exists not only *in utero* but also within a matrix of anticipations, predispositions, parental personalities, social communities, and the wider gestalt of the world condition. The milieu into which the child is born is influenced by, and in turn will come to influence, the child. Consequently, this study seeks to address simultaneously the psychological issues of integration and differentiation of identity. It views the mother-infant dyad, at once, as a unity, as two individuals together, and as two individuals imbedded within a larger family and social network.

Precursors of this reciprocal interaction between the mother and neonate are found in the expectant woman's experience of pregnancy and in her imaginings about her unborn child. Interlocking physiological processes between mother and fetus are paralleled by psychological ones. As her body expands to accommodate the growth of her fetus, so the expectant mother finds her psychic and affective life altering to include another person. Along with changes in her relationships to others, brought about by the awareness of an impending new arrival, the pregnant woman often experiences important shifts in her internal orientation. The heightened emotional sensitivities of pregnancy and the tendency toward diminished interest in external concerns increase a woman's awareness of subtle undercurrents in herself, the discovery of which may provoke anxiety or distress.

The increased complexity of relationships in the external family situation is paralleled by an increased complexity of internal object relations. Somehow a place must be prepared for an as yet unknown person on both intrapsychic and interpersonal levels. Part of this preparation may occur via moods which leave the expectant mother feeling herself alternately as adult—integrated and competent—and as infant—re-gressed, helpless, and under the sway of potentially disintegrative forces.

The fluidity of this internal state predisposes the mother to an em-pathic relationship with her newborn infant who also experiences wide fluctuations in mood and an unstable sense of self. A woman's urge to examine and consolidate her resources in response to these shifts in the internal balance of her personality may call forth submerged parental imagos, dormant until precipitated by the anticipation of becoming a par-ent herself. With the creation of one's own family, perceptions of and identifications with one's parents may change, become better integrated or differentiated. Yet questions about one's capacity to be different from one's own parents may also arise as a woman experiences herself in the mothering role for the first time. In turn, these internal concerns operate to increase or diminish the precedence of the marital bond over ties to one's family of origin.

The dramatic physical changes of pregnancy focus a woman's atten-tion on her body in ways reminiscent of adolescence or early childhood. Discomfort, pain, headaches, nausea, weight gain, and other symptoms may leave a woman feeling out of control or beseiged by her body in unpredictable and anxiety-provoking ways. The emotional turmoil which can be a part of this time has generally been considered an artifact of pregnancy's hormonal shifts, been attributed to women's "innate emo-tional nature," or been ascribed to the specific psychopathology of indi-vidual women. Consequently, physical symptomatology, level of anxiety, neuroticism, or introversion have usually been the preferred variables investigated in efforts to understand pregnancy.

The actual nature of women's anxieties or preoccupations during pregnancy has received remarkably little attention. What is it that women worry about when they are pregnant? This study suggests that, if one considers the realistic physical hazards of pregnancy and the emotional complexities of introducing another person into the family constellation, these anxieties may not only be more comprehensible, but may be seen to serve important psychological functions.

Pregnancy as an event of psychological import was first recognized by women psychoanalysts such as Helene Deutsch (1945), Grete Bibring (1961), and Therese Benedek (1952, 1959). They emphasized that preg-nancy and motherhood have developmental significance in the lives of women and represent a maturational sequence which diverges from the masculine pattern taken as the norm. Yet many issues in regard to preg-nancy remain unexplored, particularly in terms of how women define this experience for themselves. Most developmental perspectives, while em-phasizing the psychological sequelae of pregnancy, suffer to some extent from their own bias. Female maturity becomes translated into satisfactory adaptation to the maternal role. What is overlooked is that maternity is imbedded within a social context which shapes the unfolding of that role.

Today's pregnant woman finds herself in a phylogenetically new situation. The advent of effective and readily available contraceptives, the contemporary trend of sexual relationships of undefined commitment or duration, and the ready availability and convenience of abortion all have profoundly changed the emotional, psychological, and biological climate in which pregnancy occurs. Concurrent with these events, a woman's place in the world is undergoing transformation. While men have retained fairly well-defined roles, women are now expected to juggle multiple roles at once. Integrating a professional life with the desire for children is especially difficult, given the level of commitment needed to succeed at either of these often conflicting enterprises.

Pressures to limit population growth, coupled with the feminist movement's criticism of the motherhood mystique, have added to the devaluation of the mothering role in American society. The admiration and support accorded a mother or prospective mother in earlier societies has given way to an ambivalent state where concerns about pregnancy interrupting a woman's career offset respect for her new standing as a mother. These extrinsic factors influencing a woman's views of herself as a prospective mother are mirrored intrapsychically. There is a struggle for rapprochement between the identity for which the woman has prepared herself, through education and aspiration in the working world, and the identity for which nature has biologically and psychologically prepared her—that of mother.

An individual's resolution of this complex dilemma may be quite protracted, and increasingly, professional women are postponing their first child until the last possible moment—delivering their firstborn in their late 30's or even early 40's. The impact of such social trends is reflected in the intrapsychic struggles of individuals and, of course, these struggles are in turn projected back into society at large.

It is necessary, therefore, to consider not only the fetus or the woman, or even the couple as the heuristic focus of this study, but also the interaction of each of these with one another and within the overall societal context. The personal integration of social and intrapsychic dichotomies may be considered part of the "work" of pregnancy. In contemporary American society, "motherhood" is charged with stereotyped images of endless patience, self-sacrifice, and love for all aspects of the child and the mothering role. These idealized "good mother" images exist side by side with images of the "bad mother"—who is selfish, depriving, and insensitive to her child's needs. These split images exist without consideration for such social realities as the effect on the mother of isolation, low status attached to being a housewife, physical exhaustion, and the interruption of higher status professional involvement. Internalized images of the "good" and "bad" mother also exist in the psyche of pregnant women, reflecting both society's stereotypes and their experience of the "good" and "bad" aspects of their own mothers. What is generally lacking, both in the culture and in the experience of many expectant mothers, is some realistic assessment of the specific pleasures and frustrations of childbearing and child-rearing.

Despite being well-educated, the women in this study are a case in point. They began pregnancy with little knowledge of what was actually involved. The extent of the physical and emotional changes they underwent was at times a source of surprise and distress. While this uninformed state was buffered as pregnancy progressed by reading and self-education, the initial ignorance of these women is in keeping with findings of other studies on pregnancy (Leifer, 1980; Newton, 1973). These studies indicate that lack of knowledge about pregnancy is pervasive in contemporary society; more common are negative valuations of pregnancy as a passive, undesirable, alien state which is a regrettable, though inevitable, part of having a child.

At the beginning of the interviewing process, the women in this study recalled their previous lack of interest in pregnancy, and to a lesser extent in motherhood itself, although they all felt that having a child was something they wanted as part of their life experience. As their pregnancies progressed, they tended to integrate these views with a more positive appreciation of pregnancy as an active phase heralding important shifts in their lives and their primary relationships. Much of their worrying about themselves, their unborn child, their husbands, and others was a matter of coming to grips with the central dynamics of their lives and an emerging sense of themselves as "good-enough" mothers. Sometimes this was accompanied by the recognition that they had received "good-enough," if not always optimal, mothering themselves. Sometimes it yielded a definite sense of being different from their own and other mothers. In every case the changes were felt to be profound and important, signaling a new developmental line in the expectant mother's sense of herself as an individual and in her relations with others.

Theorists of adult development view personality not as an entity fixed in adolescence, but as a fluid process amenable to growth throughout the life cycle. Milestones such as marriage, parenthood, and retirement are seen as opportunities for continued maturation. The concept of pregnancy and parenthood as a significant life stage has been advanced by theorists such as Erikson (1959), Deutsch (1945), and Caplan (1962). Here too, however, the research suffers from an inclination to view feminine development basically as a variation of male-determined stages of life, neglecting pregnancy and motherhood as decisive stages in their own right.

There is even less knowledge about the significance pregnancy holds for women at different stages in life. Pregnancy and motherhood are experienced differently by women who are older, and presumably more settled in their lives, than by younger women still forming an adult identity. In Steinhoff's (1978) study, young women who had used contraception or aborted an unplanned pregnancy tended to be future-oriented with high expectations for themselves and the children they intended to have later. On the other hand, women who opted for motherhood in their late teens or early 20s felt that having a baby would give them a sense of importance and adult status they did not yet possess.

The configuration of personality, marital status, work aspirations, and preparation for parenthood is, obviously, different in the 30s from that in the 20s and affects the way pregnancy is viewed. Women in the present study felt that a certain level of maturity and stability had to be achieved before they could in good conscience become mothers. For them, the decision to experience pregnancy and bear a child rested on an internal sense that they were now ready to give expression to a side of themselves previously deferred. Their desire for maturity and stability as prerequisites for having a child involved satisfying educational, professional, and emotional goals. Recognition of the "biological clock" was, thus, only one among a number of factors.

The interaction of work and career matters with the urge to bear children and the practicalities of raising a family are examined in this study. In particular, the degree to which working outside the home and raising a family complement and/or interfere with one another is examined. The influence of work as an environmental ("social") variable on the pregnant woman, her mentation, and emotions is studied to determined the co-influence of work and childbearing. Childbearing has an intrinsic structure, commencing at conception, which may or may not "fit" with extrinsic structures imposed by the working world. These two structuring variables are, in one way or another, integrated in the woman's experience of herself as she becomes a mother.

Hypotheses regarding the ego-building effect of work are also advanced. While Freud posited that work anchors the ego in a stable matrix of reality, it may be that pregnancy has precisely the opposite effect, taking the woman deeper into her own world of subjective "reality" and fantasies about herself and child. Melanie Klein (1937) suggested that men's ambitiousness in work is a sublimation of their envy of the womb, with its biological potential for creation and nurturance of life. To what extent can this mechanism be seen in the ambitions of a pregnant woman? Is her libido divided between her pregnancy and her work, or is interest in one sacrificed at the expense of the other?

A woman's attitudes about her pregnancy may express some of these libidinal flows. In the present study clues are sought regarding ways in which women's professional goals and experiences may influence what they want and experience in childbearing. Connections between drives and impulses in personal and professional areas of these women's lives are inferred from the flow of their associations, thoughts, feelings, fantasies, and experiences during pregnancy.

The bringing into being of a human infant is seen as an extended process of finely interwoven factors. The pregnancy reorganizes, and at the same time is organized by the social, historical, and psychological formations surrounding the mother. Maternal feeling and a sense of self as mother emerge out of the integration of this wealth of intrapsychic and experiential material.

1

Historical Background

Overview

Historically, pregnancy and its role in a woman's development have been defined in different ways. Both cultural preoccupations and prevailing perceptions of male/female roles are reflected in these views. Two basic underlying positions can be distinguished. The one considers pregnancy as passive: an anticipatory prelude to motherhood in which gestation unfolds mechanically and little change occurs in the mother's personality. This portrays the woman stereotypically, as passive, reactive, lacking in influence, being perhaps invaded against her nature by the active male principle which initiates the development of the embryo.

This view perhaps owes something to the image of millions of sperm entering the womb in search of the ovum. On finding an egg, several sperm discharge their sperm lysins against the surface of the helpless ovum. These dissolve the egg membrane locally and allow one sperm to enter and fertilize the ovum, initiating gestation. Of course, closer analysis refutes this simplistic view of fertilization even at the simplest physiological level. The egg is highly prepared for the approach of the sperm, and the cytoplasm of the egg reaches out to envelop and "swallow" the sperm into the egg. Simultaneously, specialized cells on the surface of the ovum swell and explode to form the fertilization membrane which both keeps other sperm out and traps the swallowed sperm inside. Further intraovular processes actually guide the sperm to its destiny of fusion with the X chromosomes in the ovum (Balinsky, 1970). It is thus perhaps fair to speak of the egg as "lying in wait" for the approaching sperm.

The other point of view sees pregnancy as an active, transforming event in a woman's life. By this event something about the woman is forever changed. This approach reflects more the infinitely complex physiological and psychological active readiness of the woman for pregnancy: for the creation, embryonic development, gestation, delivery, and nurturance of a child. In this study the actual processes of pregnancy will be examined to portray the woman's activity and responsiveness to the phenomenon of her own first pregnancy.

Primitive Societies

The understanding of human reproduction in primitive cultures often linked pregnancy with belief in the supernatural. The male role in procreation was not always recognized, and the female role was considered primary. The belief that pregnancy came as a result of possession by spirits was widespread. In *The Sexual Life of Savages,* Malinowski (1929) describes how the Trobriand Islanders, while aware that a virgin could not conceive, nonetheless maintained that pregnancy occurred only when a woman was invaded by ancestral spirits symbolized in the totem animal. Freud (1913), in *Totem and Taboo,* notes similar beliefs but interprets such beliefs as a function of denial rather than ignorance. He suggests that denial served defensive purposes by placing the responsibility for survival of the tribe on the totem animal rather than on the individual male.

The couvade (from the French *couver,* meaning to hatch) is an elaborate ritual in which men simulate the delivery of a child themselves by taking to their beds and crying out in pain during a woman's confinement. The custom has been noted since early antiquity and is still practiced by males in many preliterate societies today (Mead, 1949). There are various interpretations of its meaning, but the association of the couvade with societies in transition from matriarchal to patriarchal social organization has generally led to its being thought of as one of the means by which men gradually take over the governing functions of women. It is also possible that the couvade may have constituted a way of managing the awe and envy of the female aroused by her central role in pregnancy and childbirth. By providing the father with an active, though ritualized, part in the birth process, the couvade both establishes paternity and accords a man the same status after the ritual birth as a postpartum female. Yet the implication of the couvade remains; the act of giving birth, a female function, is more highly valued than the act of impregnation. Fatherhood is thus demonstrated by taking on maternal characteristics.

The primacy of the female reproductive function in primitive cultures was often venerated by worship of the female in her maternal form. Woman as simultaneous vessel and giver of life was most often depicted as a pregnant woman or as a woman with a newborn child (Neumann, 1955). Both Bachofen (1967) and Briffault (1927) point out that this worship of the female as pregnant or as mother generally occurs in matriarchal societies where the male role in sexual reproduction is not well understood or not emphasized. Recognition of the male role, on the other hand, appears to correlate with a shift from matriarchal to patriarchal social organization. In patriarchal societies, the male role in reproduction is emphasized while the female role is seen as secondary. In this context, pregnancy becomes a waiting period with the female as a passive host to an active male seed. This interaction between biological and social/psychological definitions of male and female roles continued to play a part in subsequent views about pregnancy.

Prescientific and Classical Ideas

Differing views concerning the active or passive nature of pregnancy co-existed in classical times. Aristotle, for instance, extended his philosophical preoccupations with "form" and "substance" to the realm of human reproduction. He introduced the idea of an active creative principle, which was male (form), and a passive principle, which was female (substance). In this way, he felt, the fetus was built up from the union of the sperm and the menstrual blood withheld during gestation (Briffault, 1927). Hippocrates held a similar view, though he differentiated the male seed into two kinds, the "weak" seed which produced a female and the "strong" seed which produced a male.

In contrast to this line of thinking which viewed the woman as merely the soil for the male seed, and which was not interested in the effects of pregnancy on the mother, numerous myths of this period present pregnancy and childbirth as a female mystery of transformation. The Eleusian Mysteries, for example, based on the Demeter-Persephone myth, celebrated the transformation of Persephone the maiden, into Demeter the mother, via the childbearing experience (Kerenyi, 1949; Jung, 1949). Implicit in the myth is the assumption that woman as mother is different from woman as maiden. Transmutation of one to the other occurs through pregnancy and childbirth.

The myth recounts the rape of Persephone, the primordial maiden, by Hades, lord of the underworld. When Demeter, Persephone's mother, hears of the rape, she searches everywhere, but without success, for her daughter. Her grief over the loss of her daughter is so great that Demeter, goddess of the earth and the harvest, can no longer perform her functions. As a result, the fertility of the fields is interrupted and everything becomes barren. This catastrophe bends even Zeus to her will, and Demeter is eventually reunited with her daughter, but only for a limited time each year. Persephone has eaten some pomegranate seeds while in the underworld, so must remain part of the year with her husband in the underworld where she gives birth to a child of her own.

As maiden, Persephone belongs to her mother. Her separation from her mother begins with her rape or impregnation by Hades, who carries her off and marries her. When she returns to her mother, Persephone is no longer the same. She has become a mother herself. Yet she returns to Demeter and remains partially connected to her. The strength of the mother-daughter tie between Demeter and Persephone, as well as the transformation of Persephone, hinges on their shared experience as women. Demeter was herself raped by Poseidon when she became mother of Persephone. The emphasis on female experience in this myth specifically ties together the transformation of maiden into mother, with the rebirth of the mother via the return of the maiden. Commenting on the Demeter-Persephone myth, Jung (1949) writes:

> The psyche pre-existent to consciousness (e.g., in the child) participates in the ma-ternal psyche on the one hand, while on the other it reaches across to the daughter psyche. We could therefore say that every mother contains her daughter in herself and every daughter her mother, and that every woman extends backwards into her mother and forwards into her daughter. (p. 162)

The connection between women, then, is their capacity to bear children, to bear each other as it were. Childbearing, in turn, changes something about a woman. In the myth, one finds various aspects of feminine experience personified. There is Persephone, the unmarried maiden; Persephone, the married and impregnated woman; Demeter, the mother with child and Demeter, the mother without her child. Each of these has different characteristics and illustrates different phases in a woman's development from maiden to mother.

Early Scientific Ideas

Debate about the respective active or passive nature of a woman's role in gestation continued throughout the seventeenth and eighteenth centuries. The ontogenetic development of animals was explained by the theory of preformation. Before the discovery of spermatozoa, this theory supposed that the embryo, and therefore indirectly the future animal as well, already existed preformed in the egg. When spermatozoa were discovered in 1677, however, the relative significance of the ova and the spermatozoa were reevaluated (Balinsky, 1970). Two rival schools resulted, each arguing in favor of either the ova or the spermatozoa as the carrier of the preformed embryo. The ovists claimed that the preformed embryo resided in the egg and that the spermatozoa were merely parasites living in the seminal fluid. The animalculists (from the word *animalcule*, which was the name given to spermatozoa), on the other hand, insisted that the embryo was preformed in the spermatozoon and that the egg only provided the nutrition for its development. In 1694, a Dutchman, Hartsaker, drew a picture of the "homunculus," or "little person," hidden in the spermatozoon (de Beauvoir, 1952). This was in keeping with the earlier Aristotelian notion that the woman was simply the passive nourisher of a living, dynamic principle.

While not universally accepted, the views of the ovists and animalculists were discussed into the nineteenth century. New discoveries in the study of embryology in the nineteenth century, particularly Roux's experiments with egg cleavage in the frog in the late 1800's (Balinsky, 1970), led to the abandonment of the theory of preformation. By 1883 the details of the union of the nuclei of the two gametes, egg and sperm, within the fertilized ovum were first worked out by the Belgian zoologist van Beneden (de Beauvior, 1952). The biologically equal value of the nuclei of the two gametes, however, did little to change the view that gestation was essentially a passive condition in which the female remained static while nurturing an active principle within her.

Psychoanalytic and Other Contributions

The emergence of psychoanalytic thinking in the early 1900's stimulated an elaboration of female psychology (Freud, 1905). Here, pregnancy was viewed as a central expression of female sexuality and the natural outcome of mature feminine development (Deutsch, 1949). The exact ways in which feminine development was affected, however, were not specifically delineated, but were subsumed under the concept of "motherliness" (Deutsch, 1949). This perspective is not unlike that dramatized in myths. In both cases, pregnancy was perceived as an event of transformative significance for women, yet the actual processes by which the "transformation" was accomplished were not clarified. The transformation was linked to unconscious processes. It occurred in darkness, in the underworld of experience or, in psychoanalytic terms, in the unconscious. Its visible manifestation was in the relation of mother and child. In other words, while pregnancy remained something of a mystery, it was clear that childbirth produces not only a child, but also a mother.

With increasing emphasis on female psychology, fresh perspectives with regard to pregnancy emerged, particularly in its normal manifestations. Initial psychosomatic interpretations (Benedek, 1959) were followed by theoretical formulations of pregnancy as a developmental crisis leading to a higher maturational integration of the personality (Bibring, 1959; Bibring et al., 1961; Menninger, 1943). The concepts of developmental crisis and enhanced personality integration suggest that pregnancy is potentially an integrating principle in female psychology, and support the view that parturition is transformative in character.

More recently, widespread changes in women's roles and the increase in education and professional opportunities for women have produced new trends in childbearing patterns (Glick, 1977). Scientific advances in contraception and the liberalization of abortion have posed complex new social, psychological, and medical questions for mothers-to-be: what Caryl Rivers (1975) has called the "new anxiety of motherhood." More and more women are delaying childbearing in favor of education, professional advancement, or simply to give themselves more time to "feel ready" (Colman, 1978). It may be that the more elective nature of pregnancy will eventually require women to work out a new relationship to this event in their lives. It is no longer a foregone conclusion that all women will wish to become pregnant when they marry or simply because they reach adulthood.

These changes, together with continuing demands from the women's movement for more adequate theories of feminine development, have focused renewed interest on pregnancy and its social and psychological consequences in women's lives. Traditional standards of medical obstetrics and prenatal care have been challenged on grounds of their questionable effects on mother and child alike (Chertock, 1969; Verny, 1981). The values of professional development for women and the raising of children have been experienced as being most often in conflict. It is during pregnancy that these conflicting values tend to become most apparent. The course of pregnancy is generally somewhat unpredictable. Some women have more adverse reactions than others. These reactions may interfere with the best-laid plans and leave women suddenly aware of physical limits or emotional vulnerabilities to which they were previously indifferent. Caught in the crosscurrents of conflicting values, and separated from the traditional support of extended family by a highly mobile society, many pregnant women feel isolated and ambivalent as they anticipate becoming mothers (Rivers, 1975).

While much has been learned in the past few decades about the physiology of pregnancy, its psychology has remained more elusive (Benedek, 1970; Colman, 1971). The new fields of prenatal psychology, fetology, and psycho-obstetrics, which are the result of scientific efforts to understand the origins of life, have been primarily concerned with investigating the nature of fetal life. Some crucial emotional, as well as physiological links which bind a woman and her unborn child together have come to light in the process. These indicate that a woman's feelings about her pregnancy may actually play a vital role in fetal development (Sontag, 1966; Verny, 1981). Much emphasis has been placed in recent years on the process of emotional attachment, or bonding, which takes place between mother and infant after birth. Less attention has been given to the process of attachment which occurs between a mother and her unborn child during pregnancy. The psychology of pregnancy may offer important clues in understanding this process better. A woman's feelings about herself and her fantasies about her unborn child may constitute the groundwork for her later relationships with her child.

Except for scattered accounts of particular case histories in the psychoanalytic literature, little attention has been paid to the subjective experience of pregnancy in the individual lives of women who are not under psychiatric care. Nor has much attention been paid in the literature to the interplay between aspects of adult development and the age at which pregnancy occurs. The discovery that there are developmental periods over the life course (Gould, 1978; Levinson et al., 1978; Sheehy, 1974) and the recent changes in childbearing patterns now raise questions which remain to be addressed. In what way age shapes a woman's subjective experience of a first pregnancy is still largely unknown.

Modern obstetrics has greatly reduced the physical dangers of pregnancy, but what about the psyche of the pregnant woman? Are there psychological tasks or dilemmas to be negotiated, which were previously channeled through rituals or through social conventions, that traditionally accorded pregnant women special privileges, guarded them from sudden frights, or warded off the malevolent "evil eye" throughout pregnancy?

This study, by documenting and analyzing the subjective experience of a first pregnancy for four women, elucidates how a woman defines this experience for herself. Does she experience herself differently? What are her hopes and fears, her dreams and fantasies, during this time? It is from this understanding of how a woman experiences the changes occurring within her that this study begins to identify the physical, psychological, and social factors which come together in the overall experience of pregnancy. Building on the work of earlier theorists who suggest that pregnancy leads to "higher maturational integration of the personality" (Bibring, 1959; Bibring et al., 1961), the effects of pregnancy as an integrating principle of female psychology will thus be elaborated. This study of four highly educated women in their early 30's will allow this elaboration with special reference to issues in adult development.

2

Review of the Literature

Overview

Contemporary literature on pregnancy and childbirth falls into three main categories—medical, psychoanalytic, and psychological. The medical literature concerns itself with the description and classification of the frequency and treatment of specific difficulties encountered in connection with childbearing.

Psychoanalytic studies based on a limited number of cases, most often of women who were or became pregnant while in analysis, study childbearing as an aspect of female sexuality. Therese Benedek (1959), for example, describes the different feeling states during pregnancy which accompany psychological difficulties and hormonal changes. Other psychoanalytic writers, also drawing on their clinical experience, such as Helene Deutsch in her *Psychology of Women* (1944), discuss pregnancy and childbirth in more theoretical terms. Acceptance of the maternal role is symbolized by healthy adjustment to pregnancy and infant care. This constitutes the central task of psychosexual feminine maturity.

Aside from medical and psychoanalytic literature, there are a number of more specifically psychological studies which utilize rigorous methodologies to investigate different personality variables as they relate to pregnancy. Two different positions which underlie the many variations in research on pregnancy and childbirth need to be distinguished. These are reminiscent of the historical debate over the woman's active or passive role in parturition. One views pregnancy as a "hurdle" (Breen, 1975) or temporary illness from which a woman recovers when she returns to her prepregnancy state more or less unchanged. The other position, and the one adopted in the present study, assumes that the experience of pregnancy is "developmental," i.e., pregnancy involves a woman in a process from which she emerges in some way significantly different from her previous self.

A review of the more contemporary literature follows. Drawing on material from all three categories, it demonstrates the present limited state of knowledge and of methodology to derive knowledge concerning a woman's experience of a first pregnancy.

Pregnancy as Illness: The Hurdle Perspective

Studies which view pregnancy as a "hurdle" to be negotiated consider a healthy outcome to consist of a simple return to the prepregnancy state. Changes accompanying pregnancy are seen as transient in spite of their frequent disorganizing impact on the personality. "Weak" or "neurotic" egos may respond to pregnancy with pathological reactions, but the "normal" woman experiences pregnancy only as a temporary disruption of her previous equilibrium. Implicit in this thinking is the notion of pregnancy as an illness from which a woman may or may not recover (Lomas, 1973).

Using the Maudsley Personality Inventory, Chapple and Furneaux (1964) found that women who scored high on neuroticism tended to become more introverted as pregnancy progressed. Women who scored low on neuroticism did not show significant fluctuation in their introversion scores. Both groups returned to previous scores after childbirth. The authors conclude from this that pregnancy acts as a "non-specific" stress to which response varies according to the woman's initial personality. In other words, there is little which can be said about changes occurring in pregnancy except that a woman's prepregnancy personality has some bearing on how disruptive she finds the experience. Ultimately, according to this way of thinking, once pregnancy ends, its effects also disappear. Overlooked in this conclusion is the fact that an effect of pregnancy which does not disappear is the birth of a child.

Similarly, Jarrahi-Zadek et al. (1969) used the Cattell Neuroticism Scale Questionnaire to establish that pregnancy is accompanied by an "increased level of neuroticism," particularly in the third trimester and the first week postpartum. The authors considered the increased level of neuroticism a general, or normal, feature of pregnancy and delivery due to either the anticipated or actual difficulty of childbirth.

These and other studies (Kear-Colwell, 1965; Treadway et al., 1969) confirm that pregnancy is a time of emotional upheaval. Increased levels of neuroticism seem to be present regardless of age, social class, type of delivery, or length of labor. Yet terms referring to "increased neuroticism," and the use of questionnaire scales devised to distinguish psychiatric from nonpsychiatric patients imply that pregnancy is indeed an illness rather than a developmental process.

Perhaps the most frequently used concept to describe the psychological condition of women who experience obstetric complications is that of anxiety. One study (Davids, 1962) used a questionnaire to show that high anxiety during pregnancy correlated with an increase in abnormal delivery room records. Women with low anxiety scores during pregnancy tended to have normal deliveries. Anxiety scores after delivery were the same for both groups. In contrast, Brown (1964), using the same questionnaire but the narrower criterion of length of labor, was unable to establish a relationship between level of expressed anxiety and duration of labor.

These types of discrepancies in results have led some authors to introduce the idea of suppression of emotion. Cramond (1954), for example, found no relation between difficulty of labor and anxiety expressed postpartum. He felt, however, that women who had experienced difficulties tended to repress emotions. He inferred this tendency by reviewing previous medical records to reveal a higher incidence of psychosomatic symptoms such as peptic ulcers in women who had difficult labors but did not express anxiety overtly. The tendency to inhibit the expression of fears in women suffering from difficult labor has been suggested by other authors as well (Jeffcoate, 1955; Watson, 1959).

These studies illustrate the problem of distinguishing between anxiety which is repressed (unconscious) and anxiety which is suppressed (consciously withheld from the researcher). Women who represss anxiety remain genuinely unconscious of their fears which may be expressed via other channels such as psychosomatic symptomatology. Women who suppress emotions may simply not express their fears overtly, even though they are aware of them, because of their desire to appear more in control of themselves. Such distinctions are important where research relies on questionnaires since they may play a significant part in the reliability of the results.

Kogan (1968) in particular, has pointed out the problems of using questionnaires and standardized scales because of their insensitivity to subtle changes in specific groups. Kogan came to this conclusion as a result of his study of unwed mothers. When he analyzed the results obtained via questionnaire according to the standardized scales in use for his instrument, he did not find women describing themselves as significantly changed by the experience of pregnancy. When he reanalyzed his results regrouping items and using factor analysis, however, it was possible to identify important changes. In this instance, women described themselves as becoming more self-reliant, warmer, and less self-indulgent after parturition.

In some cases, attempts have been made to correlate pathological reactions during pregnancy with different types of psychopathology. Using personality questionnaires such as the MMPI, McDonald (1968) and Ringrose (1961) found that women who had prenatal or postnatal difficulties were more likely to have abnormal scores. Yet results show little beyond the fact that women who were presented with difficulties in pregnancy and childbirth appear more disturbed on a questionnaire.

These studies are consonant with the concept of pregnancy as a hurdle. The measures used are designed to assess fairly stable personality attributes and are not attuned to subtle changes over time. For the most part, they say that pregnancy can produce pathological reactions in anxious or neurotic women while the status quo is maintained in normal women.

The question remains as to how helpful it is to describe women who experience difficulties during pregnancy as neurotic. Does this say anything important about how women experience this event in their lives? And what about normal women? It appears from Kogan's study with unwed mothers that even these women, pregnant in less than favorable circumstances, experienced themselves differently after pregnancy and delivery. How then might women in favorable circumstances understand their experience? Also, if pregnancy is accompanied by emotional upheaval, as seems clear from studies which show an increased level of neuroticism, do women who are older experience this in specific ways?

Pregnancy: A Developmental Perspective

In 1931, Freud pointed out the significance of woman's double sexual role. In keeping with his orientation to instinctual drives, his paper "Female Sexuality" discusses the psychosexual aspects of the necessity to, first, attract a man and have a sexual relationship with him and, second, produce children and assume the mothering role. Psychological consequences of these events for female identity are related in the first instance to feelings of sexual desirability and various facets of the wifely role and in the second instance to maternal attributes expressed by the capacity to be a loving, nurturing person.

While these aspects of female sexuality are interrelated, success in one area may not always be accompanied by success in the other; indeed, one may compensate for the other. Social, cultural, and environmental factors have significant bearing on the evolution of either role, as do individual life histories and psychological factors. In the case of pregnancy, every society provides women with "models" of pregnancy, birth, and mother-child relations. Successful adoption of these models is likely to correspond with successful adjustment to pregnancy and motherhood. The concept of "cultural models" comes from cross-cultural research by Mead and Newton (1962), who found that symptoms generally associated with pregnancy and even the experience of pain in childbirth vary widely in different cultures, although there are natural limits imposed by what is biologically possible and physiologically normal. The diversity of experience which they document testifies to the fact that pregnancy and the experience of motherhood it engenders are both multifaceted and elaborated out of interwoven cultural, physical, and psychological factors.

Pregnancy, like puberty, is a biosocial event which elicits patterned behavior and sets in motion an evolving process at both somatic and psychological levels. It is a period which Grete Bibring (1961) has defined as containing an element of crisis. This is particularly evident in first pregnancies where the woman passes from the condition of childlessness to parenthood. Here, crisis is not considered as pathology but in the more general sense of connoting a decisive stage in the course of events.

Whereas Freud's theoretical system viewed childbearing as a compensatory development for acceptance of the feminine role—child equals penis—(1925), later theorists such as Deutsch (1944), Horney (1926), Benedek (1959), and Bibring (1961) studied female psychosexual development as a maturational sequence in its own right. Retaining Freud's concept of instinctual drives, Deutsch (1944) nonetheless rejected his compensatory concept of femininity. According to Deutsch (1944), the feminine woman is characterized by:

> a harmonious interplay between narcissistic tendencies and masochistic readiness for painful giving and loving. In the motherly woman, the narcissistic wish to be loved is metamorphosed. (Vol. 2, p. 17)

Deutsch did emphasize that motherliness is an inherent aspect of the feminine character even in women who have never borne a child, but she continued to feel that the full potentialities of this quality were most finally realized by the experience of pregnancy. Specifically, she felt that pregnancy allows a woman to move beyond her own infantile dependencies and her narcissistic adolescent preoccupation with her own seductiveness. In reversing the original mother-child symbiosis, pregnancy also revives past conflicts over separation-individuation and may renew concern with issues of identity. Gradually, there occurs a metamorphosis, or transfer of interest from the outside of the body (narcissistic) to its inner contents (the baby). Deutsch stressed the active components in feminine development, relating these specifically to changes occurring in women as a result of pregnancy and motherhood.

Horney (1967), likewise, challenged Freud's negative valuation of feminine development and particularly emphasized the positive aspects of femininity represented in motherhood.

In her classic studies of psychosexual functions in women, Benedek (1952, 1959) posits that feminine maturation occurs through step-by-step identification with the mother. Menarche is the start of the reproductive function, and pregnancy is the beginning of mature womanhood with respect to responsibility for the life of another being. Benedek is careful to distinguish the importance of the psychological dimension in human mothering behavior. She writes:

> the slow ontogenic maturation of human offspring necessitated the evolution of social structures which, in turn, allow for and require a broad range of modifications in mothering behavior. It is only the human female whose mothering behavior has two resources: One is, as in any creature, rooted in her physiology; the other evolves as an expression of her personality. (1970, p. 153)

Bibring (1961), who first introduced the concept of pregnancy as a maturational crisis, also considers it as a period of increased libidinal tasks, a time of acute disequilibrium marked by disturbed thinking processes and the emergence of repressed material reminiscent of borderline conditions. These features are seen as symptomatic of internal psychological reorganization which becomes stabilized in the course of early mother-infant interaction.

In this respect it is important to emphasize the mutually interactive process of mother and child. Loesch and Greenberg (1962), for example, contend that pregnancy by itself is not necessarily developmental. They feel that certain processes and internal events must be mobilized if pregnancy is to serve as a developmental period. In their study, unmarried subjects who gave their babies up for adoption showed little evidence of psychological change. Bibring and Rubin (1967) concur with this point of view. They feel that the birth of the baby consolidates the changes promoted during pregnancy.

While it is risky to transpose from animal studies to human behavior, the work of comparative psychologists Rosenblatt and Lehrmann (1963) substantiates the importance of a mutually interactive process in the evolution of maternal response. In their study of mother-young synchrony in rats, they observed that hormonal changes occurring shortly before delivery institute maternal behavior which has a fixed and automatic pattern. The newborn plays an active part in stabilizing this pattern. Absence of suckling for four days postpartum is followed by the disappearance of mothering behavior which subsequent suckling cannot re-evoke.

More recent research in the field of prenatal psychology suggests a similar interactive process may occur even before birth in the form of intrauterine bonding (Verny, 1981). An example of this is Stirnimann's

(1978) study of sleep patterns in neonates. In his study, he correlated the sleep patterns of neonates with those of their mothers prior to delivery. He discovered that a child's sleeping patterns are set months before, *in utero*, by his mother, demonstrating that in the months preceding birth, mother and child already begin to mesh their rhythms and responses to each other. Other studies by Lukesch (1975) and Rottman (1974) demonstrate the significance of maternal attitudes during pregnancy for the well-being of both mother and child. Both studies show that children of accepting mothers, who looked forward to having a family, were much healthier emotionally and physically at birth and afterward than offspring of rejecting mothers.

The importance of mother-infant interaction both *in utero* and after birth argues against the notion of pregnancy as an illness or temporary condition. Illnesses do not bring forth a child, and a child, after all, remains as a lasting effect of pregnancy. What distinguishes pregnancy further from the concept of illness is that the child, while unborn, is nevertheless already a presence in the life and imagination of the expectant mother. Unlike other fantasies she may have, her fantasies about the child she carries are attached to a living being who, once born, may or may not meet her expectations. Considerations of this type begin to change the emphasis from a purely intrapersonal basis, such as neuroticism, to one more informed by interpersonal dynamics.

Benedek's (1970) emphasis on the psychological dimension present in human reproduction is important here. While studies of pregnant women assert that the baby only becomes a living reality for the mother when the first movements occur (Bonnaud & Revault D'Allones, 1963; McConnell & Daston, 1961), clues to the significance of the child within her may find their first symbolic expression in the fantasies and dreams, the worries and anxieties an expectant mother has about herself in the initial stages of pregnancy. A variable period of adjustment to the presence of another, during which a woman becomes familiar with and imagines the child before actually experiencing the first fetal movements, would seem necessary. To date, such symbolic interactions a mother has with her "imagined child" have not been generally explored. Indeed, the origins of separation-individuation issues (Kaplan, 1978; Mahler, 1968, 1971; White, 1975) may conceivably be rooted in this earliest inception of mother-child relations which occurs first in the mental life of the expectant mother.

In addition to the mother-infant relationship, other significant relationships are influenced by the experience of pregnancy. Psychoanalytic literature refers above all to the pregnant woman's relationship with her own mother. Early experiences of love and hate, satisfaction and frustration leading to "good" and "bad" mother images color a woman's representation of herself as mother and mother-to-be. Benedek (1959) notes that the way a woman identifies herself with her own mother structures her feeling about motherhood and defines her behavior towards her own children. Positive identification with the mother as a prototype of the nurturing figure correlates with successful maturation, while depression may arise when such identification with the good mother image is impossible or problematic (Racamier, 1953, 1961). Breen (1975), on the other hand, in her study of primigravidae using repertory grids and a series of questionnaires, finds that it is primarily the integration of good and bad mother images, as opposed to simple identification with the mother, which yields a positive resolution of pregnancy and childbirth. A number of her well-adjusted women actually reconstrued the mothering role rather than identifying with their own mothers.

Redefining the mothering role for oneself in addition to identifying with one's own mother as a task of first pregnancy has begun to surface elsewhere in psychoanalytic thinking and is generally discussed in terms of a woman's ongoing involvement with separation-individuation from her own mother (Morgan, 1979; Pines, 1982). First pregnancy is seen as an opportunity to come to grips with problematic aspects of this process and thus holds out the potential for further emotional differentiation within the personality.

The marital relationship is also modified by pregnancy and parturition. The husband's reactions to becoming a father and his response to the changes in his wife are crucial as the family constellation shifts from a dyadic to a triadic one (Verny, 1981). When the dyadic system is too rigid and one of the partners cannot accept the entry of a third person into the relationship, difficulties arise (Lomas, 1959). For some women, unity with the baby inside seems to replace longing for intimacy with the husband. For others, sexual desire increases in the attempt to deal with deeper anxieties (Jessner, Weigert, & Foy, 1970). In any case, the dual aspects of the feminine role described by Freud (1931/1959) come into play at this time and may entail a rebalancing of the previous marital relationship.

The woman's relationship to the world outside the home is also changed, for childbirth involves a change of status. In some cultures the first childbirth results in a change of name for the mother (Breen, 1975). Others perceive her differently and their expectations change accordingly. Once a child is born, a woman remains a "mother" forever, in terms of what Perlman (1968) has called a "vital role," i.e., a role which extends in time and feeling and cannot be abandoned.

New conflicts over the simultaneous demands of family and work may be initiated. In her study of adolescent girls, Deutsch (1967) felt that girls who planned on both career and family were unaware of a deep and powerful conflict of emotional energy inherent in their choices. She believed that the conflict of this dual choice was basically irresolvable. Jessner, Weigert, and Foy (1970) are more optimistic in their view. While recognizing the difficulties of divided commitment, they conclude:

> the compromise allows these young [working] mothers the experience of themselves as whole persons and allows a genuine enjoyment of their children without burdening their offspring with resentment or expecting them to compensate for the sacrifice. (p. 220)

The consequences of work for the experience of pregnancy is still a debated issue. The reality is that many women today do work at professional occupations they are not willing to give up when they become mothers. Many women also continue to work during their pregnancies. How work versus nonwork figures in a woman's subjective experience of pregnancy is unclear. Existing conflicts may intensify after the child is born and the realities of infant care become evident, but during pregnancy much is still a matter of speculation or imagination on the part of the mother.

Finally, entry into the maternal role is accompanied by a number of physical changes. Satisfactory adjustment to these changes has been referred to in the literature in terms of "acceptance by the woman of her female biological role" (Breen, 1975). The physiological experience of pregnancy is ideally tied to a greater sense of psychological femininity and gives a woman a fuller awareness of her sexuality (Racamier, 1953). Consequently, a woman's feelings about her body become important at this time. A woman who denies or rejects her body will find pregnancy and motherhood difficult and conflicting. Menninger (1943) attributes physical symptoms during pregnancy to a rejection of the feminine role. Chertok et al. (1963), however, feel that physiological symptomatology results from conflict and ambivalence rather than outright rejection.

Gressot (1959) adopts a somewhat more cognitive and interpersonal approach. He suggests that symptomatology in pregnancy and pain in confinement are linked to the presence of mental conflict which results from the inability to resolve contradictory elements within the personality or, more especially, the social situation in which pregnancy occurs. He comments that the effect of preparation for childbirth is to make "certain mental reactions to childbirth mutually compatible instead of antagonistic" (p. 43).

From Menninger's or Chertok's perspective, the prevalence of physical symptoms during pregnancy would certainly suggest that ambivalence about the female role is widespread in our culture. Gressot would more likely agree with Hanford (1963), who points out that no matter how much a woman desires a child, some negative aspects inevitably surface in the process of integrating such an important event into one's life.

Pregnancy as a developmental phase includes the psychological and social consequences inherent in the changed status and the reorganization of relationships which follow parturition. Much of the literature in this area, however, is based on clinical experience with patients in psychoanalysis rather than the result of planned studies. There exists relatively little research using a holistic, intensive approach. How a woman defines and redefines her experience of pregnancy over time, for instance, is rarely addressed. For example, Breen's (1975) study of 50 women having their first babies, which comes closest to portraying the ways in which a woman construes her experience, does not detail the dreams and fantasies which contribute to making the necessary adjustments at this time, nor does it discuss the results with reference to issues of adult development. Nevertheless, her results are important because of her systematic methodology. Using interviews, data from obstetricians, and a series of repertory grids designed using Kelly's personal construct theory (1955), she set out to identify adaptive and maladaptive processes in pregnancy. Her results are complex, but she concludes:

> those women who are most adjusted to childbearing are those who are less enslaved by the experience, have more differentiated, more open appraisals of themselves and other people . . . are able to call on a good mother image with which they can identify, and do not experience themselves as passive. (1975, p. 193)

The importance of collecting systematic data on the experience of pregnancy is further underlined by Kammerer (1963). In his discussion of pain in childbirth, he advocates that only the systematic collection of fantasies and dreams in pregnancy and childbirth can provide clues to the fantasy life which underlies everyday life, gives it its true meaning, and holds a key to its understanding. It is only on this basis that he thinks working hypotheses can be reliably formulated as to the scope and developmental significance of pregnancy and childbirth in female psychology.

Yet few intensive and carefully carried out observational studies of pregnancy exist. Chertok (1966) believes that observation of even a single individual case with efforts to map out its development and trace its conflicts constitutes a unique contribution because it allows for the collection of data from which extrapolations and generalizations can be made. He feels such study is rare because it represents a new departure necessitating both lucid descriptive ability and a high degree of continuity over a fairly extended period of time. It also requires a methodology capable of reconciling the practical difficulties involved in collecting systematic information while respecting the subject's own personal feelings.

Pregnancy: The Sociocultural Perspective

The sociocultural perspective takes into account the cultural mandates of particular societies. Its concern with the diversity of experience surrounding human reproductive behavior helps clarify the biological and psychological parameters of pregnancy and childbirth. The study of these events demonstrates that culture-specific meanings and personal affective meanings combine to form the symbolic matrix which underlies the way individuals understand their experience.

Social recognition of somatic events which normally attend pregnancy and childbirth, for example, varies widely. In some cultures, morning sickness is expected of every pregnant woman, while in others it is completely ignored. In still other cultures, it is believed to occur only in first pregnancies (Mead, 1950). Where morning sickness is culturally stylized, a majority of women will exhibit the expected behavior; where it is not, more idiosyncratic patterns emerge.

Cultural expectations also modulate a woman's behavior and experience of pain in labor and delivery. Some cultures expect women to cry out and shriek, while others expect them to bear their pain in utter silence or deny the pain altogether (Mead, 1950). Working-class Jamaican women speak of depression during childbirth rather than pain. This may be, in part, because they experience their first childbirth primarily as proof of their fertility and frequently give the child to someone else to raise (Brody, 1978).

Family and marital relationships are also influenced by cultural factors. In India, for example, where the extended family allows a strong bond to develop between mother and child, a pregnant woman will spend the latter part of her pregnancy preparing a bed for her husband because the newborn will sleep with her. In contrast, in the United States, where the nexus of the emotional bond in family life tends to be the husband-wife relationship, the woman prepares a bed and a separate room for the newborn (Newman, 1978).

Cultural models of motherhood may also influence a woman's experience at this time. The Judeo-Christian ideal of the self-sacrificing mother who directs herself entirely to the needs of her child is a role many women in contemporary society have internalized but find themselves in conflict with. Such conflict can form the basis for difficulties with pregnancy and the mothering role. Gordon (1967), utilizing questionnaire results, found that two factors were associated with postpartum emotional difficulties:

a "personal insecurity factor," originating from previous life experiences, and a "role-conflict" factor. While both factors were significant, continuing difficulties postpartum were found to be more related to present-day role conflict than past experience. These results are in keeping with Gressot's (1959) feeling that the inability to synthesize contradictory elements in the intrapsychic or interpersonal sphere leads to the experience of mental conflict and increased symptomatology in pregnancy and childbirth.

Alice Rossi, in her *Transition to Parenthood* (1968), suggests that a first pregnancy is characterized by a lowering of self-esteem for women due to cultural valuation of family status. She writes:

> the possibility must be faced, and at some time researched, that women lose ground in personal development and self-esteem during the early and middle years of adulthood, whereas men gain ground in these respects during the same years. The retention of a high level of self-esteem may depend on the adequacy of earlier preparation for major adult roles in the occupational system, as it does for those women who opt to participate significantly in the work world. Training in the qualities and skills needed for family roles in contemporary society may be inadequate for both sexes, but the lowering of self-esteem occurs only among women because their primary roles are within the family. (pp. 34–35)

Rossi's comments are directed to women who follow the conventional cultural model which prescribes childbearing during the 20s. How pregnancy is experienced by women in their 30s is less clear. These women have generally developed themselves professionally and so undertake the enterprise of maternity from a different vantage point. Issues of self-esteem during pregnancy may have a different significance for these women.

Post-World War II advances in birth control technology, the rise of the women's liberation movement, and widespread social changes have influenced current trends in childbearing patterns. A recent article in the *San Francisco Examiner* (July 1981) by M. Hamilton describing the "late baby boom" suggests that women, now in their 30s, who delayed childbearing to explore other less traditional avenues of self-expression, are creating a mini baby boom as they decide to begin having children. The article also suggests that these "older" mothers experience their motherhood differently as a result of being more developed professionally and more secure emotionally. Their heightened awareness of themselves and their need to understand the events of pregnancy are reflected in their insistence on extensive preparation for childbirth and the proliferation of books on pregnancy and childcare which, according to market surveys, are most often sold to older, first-time mothers.

Whether these women will experience particular dilemmas related to "role conflict" as described by Gordon (1967) remains to be seen. Dr.

L. Scott, director of the Parenthood After Thirty Project in Berkeley, feels that many women in their 30s choose to become pregnant as a social and public expression of female adequacy and identity. Such claims bring to mind psychoanalytic suppositions that maternity involves the integration of specifically feminine aspects of the personality.

Issues in Adult Development

Life-span psychology has focused on understanding personality development during adulthood. Challenging the mental stagnation model of aging, life-span psychology has demonstrated that aging can best be defined in developmental terms (Groffman, 1970). While controversy over locating distinct periods in the adult life cycle still exists, based on arguments over variations between chronological age and psychological maturity, investigators generally seem to use some type of age designation for the period of adulthood comprising years 30 through 60 or 70 (Cameron, 1969).

Various models of development have been proposed. The foremost of these are Erikson's epigenetic eight-stage model (1963) and Levinson's (1977) notion of the evolution of different life structures through a series of alternating stable and transitional stages. In Erikson's model, each stage poses a polar conflict, the resolution of which determines development at succeeding stages. For Levinson, each period is defined by the primary developmental task necessary for restructuring the previously established life structure. Changes in life structure are the result of attempts to correct flaws or fill in gaps left by the preceding structure. Significant events such as marriage, parenthood, or divorce, however, may occur at any stage and do not define a given period per se.

For Erikson, issues in young adulthood center around identity versus identity diffusion, and intimacy versus isolation. The radius of relationships at this time moves from peer group to sexual partner and gradually constellates around family and work concerns.

Levinson breaks adulthood into four distinct periods. Young adulthood (17–45 years) roughly corresponds to the same period indicated by Erikson for the resolution of specific issues around identity and intimacy. Levinson subdivides the period of young adulthood even further, however, coming to a definition of the 20s as a "novice" stage. Both Erikson and Levinson mark entry into full adulthood as beginning at age 30. For Levinson, the 30s are preceded by the Age Thirty Transition, which he describes as a period of re-evaluation during which efforts are made to rectify flaws in the provisional adult life structure built up during the 20s.

How these issues play into a woman's experience of pregnancy is not exactly clear. It seems likely that women who become pregnant in their 30s will handle issues of identity and intimacy somewhat differently than younger women. Differences may also appear between women who are working when they become pregnant and plan to continue to work after the baby's birth, and women who are not. The shift from a dyadic couple to a triadic nuclear family may represent significant changes in the life structure these women have built up in their 20s. How smoothly the transition is made may depend, in part, on their subjective evaluation of the events of pregnancy.

Rossi (1968) has commented on the lowering of self-esteem in women during first pregnancies occurring in early adulthood (17–28) at a time when men are consolidating their identities in the highly valued sphere of professional life. But women who came to adulthood in the 1970s and 1980s have increasingly reversed this traditional pattern. Exposed to conflicting social pressures about female roles, sexuality, and reproduction, many women abandoned early motherhood and lifetime child-rearing. Instead, they focused on careers and professions. How these women experience pregnancy and childbirth may reflect aspects of identity and defensive strategies developed in their 20s. Issues of self-esteem may be different than for younger women. In fact, it has been suggested that the woman who delays her first baby until her 30s and the young, pregnant teenagers are in many ways social and psychological opposites (Hamilton, 1981).

Teenagers, for instance, become pregnant because they become sexually active without using contraceptives or without using them effectively. They are erratic in protecting themselves and frequently impatient in seeking help. They often have a confused self-image and tend not to have educational or future goals. Women who delay pregnancy are just the opposite. They tend to be independent, have a sense of self-value, and plan for their future development. They choose to make use of contraceptives and may make this choice virtually hundreds of times prior to the time conception actually takes place. When they do become pregnant, they are generally more financially secure and their lives are usually more stable.

Dr. Spock, in his *Redbook* column (September 1969) comments:

> A mother still in her teens or just out of them is emotionally less apt to be tolerant of the behavior of the child, less apt to enjoy it, just because she is too close to childhood. . . . The older woman, thoroughly secure in her maturity, can enjoy those special charms of children that are expressions of their immaturity. (p. 45)

Yet pregnancy in the 30s comes at a time which may be critical for women in terms of their career development or their relationships with men. At present, little is known about the psychological implications of pregnancy at different ages. It is possible that women who have a more defined sense of themselves may experience aspects of pregnancy as intrusive or conflicting as they attempt to balance the opposing demands of professional life and maternity. Older, educated women may also feel a greater need to articulate their experience. They may want and search for a better "fit" between their feelings about pregnancy and the kind of medical care available to them. They may consequently feel more frustrated if they cannot maintain the level of control they have come to expect of themselves. In her study of delayed childbearing, Colman (1978) states that her subjects often had mutually exclusive expectations of themselves, which sometimes led to considerable conflict when satisfaction of both ideals could not be met. She also found that the primary importance of work and established work identity served as a stabilizing influence in the face of dilemmas posed by pregnancy and early infant care.

Breen's (1975) study found that both younger and older women in her group were likely to experience difficulties. Of the 50 women she studied, only five were in their 30s. Of these five, two were in the ill-adjusted group, two in the intermediary group, and one in the well-adjusted group. Breen does not say much about the age spread of her scores other than noting the results. She does say that of her total group, 78% of the women experienced some difficulty. Because her measures were introduced at various points rather than continuous over time, she believes the actual incidence of difficulties may be even higher than her results indicate. From this she concludes that pregnancy is a state of stress and upheaval which is normal, given the prevalence of problems.

Her results agree with Dr. Spock's comments in *Redbook* (September 1969):

> When you think of it, you realize that no woman could have a totally positive attitude toward an event that permanently changes the course of her life as much as any pregnancy does. (p. 46)

Conclusion

Review of the literature distinguishes two approaches to the study of pregnancy. The pregnancy-as-illness view considers pregnancy as a hurdle to be overcome. Successful negotiation of this hurdle is seen as a return to the prepregnancy state.

The developmental approach to pregnancy views gestation as a decisive period for the fuller integration of dual aspects in the feminine sexual role. It considers that physical, social, and psychological factors converge in the formation of a maternal matrix which becomes solidified in early mother-infant interaction.

Social and cultural patterns may influence the course of pregnancy both in its symptomatology and in the role expectations engendered. Where role conflict occurs and cannot be resolved, significant emotional difficulties may follow.

Aspects of adult development may affect the individual's experience of pregnancy. Women who delay childbearing may experience particular dilemmas around issues of control and the diminution of work status. How these issues are experienced and dealt with is still uncertain.

Previous studies have used a variety of research methods, such as questionnaires, rating scales, or psychological tests supplemented by more clinical data based on one or more interviews during pregnancy. These measures have generally been introduced once or twice per trimester and once postpartum. They have been structured along specific lines. Results confirm that pregnancy is a highly significant event in a woman's life frequently accompanied by emotional upheaval. It is a biosocial event; both subjectively important and important for the wider social context in which it occurs.

While these studies specify and explore particular issues along psychological, psychosomatic, or medical dimensions, they do not answer the question of what this experience entails for the woman in detail, nor how she defines and redefines the experience for herself over time. The present study addresses these questions by its use of a clinical methodology to understand the woman's own experience of her first pregnancy.

3

Methodology

Methodological Considerations

The Present Study

This study evaluates the effects of a first pregnancy on a woman and her world through anamnestic interviews of four primigravidae, beginning soon after conception and continuing to the perinatal period. Weekly interviews, including specifically psychological material, such as dreams and fantasies, detail the phenomenology of this experience and explore the meaning of this event for the women themselves.

In spite of each woman's individual experience, certain common trends emerge, representing dynamic and developmental themes central to pregnancy and to the birth of a first child. These results are presented in chapters 4, 5, and 6. Discussion of these themes in chapter 7 is framed in the larger context of adult development, as the women participating in this study are all over 30 and pregnant for the first time. The study assumes that the pregnancy experience reflects the concerns of particular periods in adult life as well as concerns specific to pregnancy itself.

The research is informed by the following proposition: During pregnancy, a woman develops a complex, highly diversified system of symbolic relationships with her unborn child which serves to integrate both her real and imagined interactions with it. This symbolic elaboration of experience occurs whenever the expectant mother assigns meaning to the physiological changes and the emotional shifts she undergoes. The meaning she gives her experience is interpretive, integrating both physical and intrapsychic factors as well as the interactions which comprise her interpersonal world.

The study follows the stance of symbolic interactionism, which sees the human being as an acting organism who actively notes, assesses, interprets, and synthesizes the play of diverse factors within the self and within the world (Blumer, 1969). From this perspective the expectant mother not only responds, but also acts upon the play of initiating factors within her and within her environment set in motion by the physiological, psychological, and interpersonal processes involved in conception, pregnancy, and confinement. She does this by subjective interpretation and evaluation of her experience which she imbues with diverse and personally significant meanings.

The study extends this interactionist perspective into its view of development. Development at any age is seen as the result of reciprocal influences between the individual and the environment. The emergence of new attitudes, abilities, or images of the self always occurs in the context of environmental opportunities, demands, and expectations. In the words of Thomas and Chess (1980), development thus becomes "a fluid dynamic process which may reinforce, modify, or change specific psychological patterns at all age periods." They refer to this concept of development as homeodynamic, as opposed to formulations which view the interplay of organism and environment as striving toward one or another form of homeostatic equilibrium.

The study also makes use of the principles of free association and dreams elaborated by Freud as an access to depth psychological phenomena. Specifically, the study takes up the relatively neglected aspect of the mentation of the primigravida, viz., that the unconscious as well as conscious associative processes of the woman herself provide a key to the understanding of her overall response to pregnancy and parturition.

The study explores the following assumptions:

1. During a first pregnancy internal preoccupations, which in turn generate idiosyncratic defensive reactions, are emphasized. Consequently, there occurs a shift of libidinal investment from external to internal phenomena.

2. Women experience both regressive and progressive tendencies which are expressed alternately by identification with the fetus (regressive) and identification with the maternal role (progressive). Both of these tendencies complement each other and serve important adaptive functions. One fosters the development of empathy in relation to the newborn's condition of general helplessness. The other promotes feelings of adequacy in relation to the active mothering role.

3. Profound emotional changes in the woman's view of herself and her world occur, leading to changes in the economy of basic mechanisms that govern unconscious functions, e.g., object relations and mechanisms of defense.

4. New adaptive constellations of defensive and emotional processes may emerge and cystallize in the form of a different and expanded sense of self. This new adaptation or interpretation of self is tested and stabilized after the child's birth in the interplay of early mother-infant interaction.

5. Specific transformative processes occurring during a first pregnancy can be understood through investigation of the expectant mother's mentation, including unconscious material such as dreams and fantasies.

6. Issues salient to the shift from a dyadic to a triadic family constellation are anticipated during pregnancy in the form of concerns about the marital relationship and body image.

7. Efforts to reconcile or integrate internalized "good" and "bad" mother images are mobilized and may find expression in the interactions between the primigravida and her own mother.

8. Issues identified as crucial in the fourth decade of life will find their way into the experience of pregnancy during the 30s and may influence how a woman views herself and her pregnancy.

9. Women oriented toward work and professional life find the integration of work and motherhood more complex and more uncertain than anticipated. These realities first emerge during pregnancy itself.

10. The first pregnancy provides an integrating force with respect to the feminine sexual role.

The Clinical Case Study Method

This study uses a process-oriented, clinical methodology suited to a longitudinal study of pregnancy and the perinatal period. This approach allowed the women who participated to speak for themselves and ensured that areas of central importance to them arose naturally from the data.

The clinical method of investigation draws largely from case study techniques prevalent in the practice of psychoanalysis, but it also derives from participant observation methods used for other disciplines such as sociology and anthropology. It is represented in the work and writings of psychoanalysts (e.g., Erikson, 1959; Freud, 1900/1938; Jung, 1916/1945); psychologists (e.g., Bettelheim, 1969; Robert White, 1959); sociologists (e.g., Lillian Rubin, 1979); social anthropologists (e.g., Bateson, 1975; Lifton, 1976; Mead, 1949); symbolic interactionists of the discipline of sociology (e.g., Blumer, 1969; George Herbert Mead, 1934); and psychologists in the field of cognitive development (e.g., Piaget, 1959). A systematic exposition of this method is available in Ralph's volume, *The Clinical Method: A Naturalistic Phenomenological Technique for Psychology* (1976). Festinger and Katz (1953), also writing on the particular merits of case study methodology, conclude:

> The great strength of the field study is its inductive procedure, its potentiality for discovering significant variables and basic relations that would never be found if we were confined to research dictated by a hypothetical-deductive model. Thus the field study and the survey are the great protection in social science against the sterility and triviality of premature model building. (p. 75)

Theoretical formulations that identify relationships of central importance in human experience most often draw from descriptive accounts, direct observations, life histories, and field studies (Blumer, 1969). These form a body of relevant observations about how people understand their world and their actions and relationships within it. The value of such accounts lies in their singular ability to remain sensitive to the process by which people organize and give meaning to their perceptions. In this regard, Blumer (1969) notes:

> The contention that people act on the basis of the meaning of their objects has profound methodological implications. It signifies immediately that if a scholar wishes to understand the action of people it is necessary for him to see their objects as they see them. Failure to see their objects as they see them, or a substitution of his meanings of the objects for their meanings, is the gravest kind of error. It leads to setting up a fictitious world. People act towards things on the basis of the meaning these things have for them, not on the basis of the meaning these things have for the outside scholar. (pp. 50–51)

A woman's subjective experience of a first pregnancy and the ways in which she finds herself changed by it involve ongoing psychological processes which may be expressed in many conscious and unconscious ways. Themes of dynamic origin, available through dreams, fantasies, and free association, as well as more cognitive schemas used to understand one's experience, are multifaceted and complex. The methodology used to examine such material must be responsive to its complicated interwoven character. Clinical case study methodology, like the approach defined by Weiss (1968) as "holistic research," attempts to discover and describe just such systems of intricate, interrelated phenomena. Weiss also suggests that it is the thorough examination of a small sample which allows full consideration of all dimensions involved in such systems. By analyzing predesignated elements and interactions, traditional experimental research suffers from the tendency to distort the true complexity of experience. In a similar vein, Lillian Rubin (1979) maintains:

> Large-scale studies based on statistically representative samples have a place in the social sciences . . . but they cannot tap all the knowledge that is potentially available. Probability studies tell us something about social trends; but they leave us guessing about their effects on the people who must live them. For that, nothing replaces the smaller-sample qualitative research based on face-to-face interaction—research that can capture the fullness and richness of life as it is experienced by those who live it, that can teach us something about the way people interpret the world and give meaning to their lives. (p. 224)

In the present study, in-depth interviews over time created an opportunity for each subject to detail and elaborate her experience, permitting rich data, supplemented by observation, to be collected. Analysis of this material focused on the typology of pregnancy and its subjective impact on the individual women studied. Tracing the development over time of individual themes within the experience of each woman, as well as exploring these issues with each woman at similar times and in similar ways, made it possible to compare women.

Despite the obvious advantages of the clinical method in dealing with an intricate, little-explored area, however, difficulties related to interpreting detailed, highly interdigitated material remain. Specifically, as mentioned previously, the psychological developments of pregnancy may occur on both conscious and unconscious levels. Consequently, a woman's perception of her experience is subject to defensive screening. The present study acknowledges the difficulty of interpretation. It provides enough interview material and insights drawn from unconscious sources such as dreams and fantasies, however, to demonstrate the basis from which conclusions were drawn.

Subjects

Research Criteria

This study investigated a first pregnancy as it occurred within selected "normal" individuals, that is, persons who were not defined either by others or by themselves as having any particular medical, emotional or interpersonal difficulties.

Women selected for this study met specific criteria. They were all over 30 and pregnant with their first child. They were pregnant under favorable conditions where changes related to pregnancy were considered more likely to occur in a clearly identifiable manner. Difficult economic conditions, dissatisfaction with the marital relationship, or an unplanned pregnancy were all factors which might have blurred the issues under investigation. Consequently, women were chosen who, according to their self-reports, considered themselves relatively happy and satisfied with their marriages and with their decision to become pregnant. They also all made the decision to become pregnant in conjunction with their husbands' expressed desire and interest in having a child. They were economically secure and well-educated.

Four such favorably situated women were chosen. Each of them was highly educated. They were all at different levels of professional development, making it possible to examine the integration of work and maternity at different stages of career development. These criteria were set to assure the selection of women who would have some insight into unconscious processes and who would be able to articulate complex mental phenomena.

The Four Women

The following description of the four women who participated in this study is an approximation of their actual characteristics. The names are pseudonyms and identifying information is disguised.

Anna (age 31). Soft-spoken, with delicate features and a love of fine music, Anna was college educated with a graduate degree in education. She taught for a few years after finishing school but decided to stop teaching when she felt she really wanted to do something else with her life. She was still uncertain about how to redefine her work interests when she became pregnant.

Rachael (age 31). Tall and slender with an attentive manner and an easy charm, Rachael was a medical doctor working in a large hospital that served a predominantly middle-class community. She became pregnant just after finishing her residency and starting a permanent staff position.

Katherine (age 31). Energetic and reserved, Katherine was a graduate student working toward her doctorate in sociology. Interested in women's issues, she had been active in community organizations and was working part-time in a women's center when she became pregnant.

Linda (age 35). Vivacious, with lively expressions and a ready smile, Linda was also a graduate student. She was working toward her master's degree in public health when she became pregnant.

Procedures

Selection Process

Although time-limited by the nature of pregnancy, the longitudinal process-oriented approach envisaged in this study asked for considerable commitments of time and energy from expectant mothers. As a result, the selection process was seen as a time during which mutual concerns and questions could be discussed in some detail prior to entering into the more comprehensive and collaborative relationship upon which this study depended.

Initial contact with prospective subjects was followed by a personal interview to determine whether the research criteria established for subject selection could be met. This first interview also provided subjects with information about the study in terms of expected time commitment, regularity of meetings, and interest in collecting in-depth psychological material such as dreams and fantasies.

After this interview, women who met the research criteria were asked to delay making their decision to participate for one week. During this time they were asked to reflect carefully about the extent of the participation needed for this study and their willingness to engage in it. It was anticipated that the additional time allotted would allow for a more firm decision. These precautionary measures were taken to safeguard the women who chose to participate and to ensure a minimal dropout rate.

Women were selected through social networking; that is, they were recruited from the periphery of the researcher's professional and social network. Approximately 10 women were interviewed before selecting the four for this study.

Data Collection

Once selected, each woman decided where she wanted subsequent interviews to take place (home, office, elsewhere), and a regular weekly meeting time was arranged. Two women were interviewed in their homes. Of the other two women, one chose to be interviewed at her office and the other preferred the researcher's office. As their pregnancy progressed, both of these women shifted the interviews to their homes. All of the postpartum interviews were conducted in the subjects' homes.

Weekly interviews, lasting between one and two hours, were conducted. After the initial interview, which was used to establish demographic data, interviews were clinical in style, a technique which is flexible and which facilitates the emergence of material from different psychological levels. Written recordings were made at the time of each interview. Women participating in this study were assured of confidentiality and the usual safeguards concerning the use of human subjects.

In selecting subjects, attention was paid to the timing of individual pregnancies. In general, expectant mothers were interviewed serially rather than concurrently, although some overlapping was planned to maintain continuity of the interviewing of the four women as a whole. This also allowed theoretical or technical refinements which emerged in the experience of interviewing one woman to enrich study of the next woman, highlighting areas of importance or pointing to individual differences.

Each woman was encouraged to report dreams and engage in free association. She was asked to express freely whatever she had on her mind, regardless of how relevant it seemed. Incidents that occurred since the previous interview, memories of experiences at any period of life, or thoughts about others, herself, or her unborn child were expected to emerge and shed light on psychological processes important for women at this time.

Strategies for Analysis

Analysis of the data emerging out of clinical techniques focuses on preserving the uniqueness of individual experience while generating systematic concepts that hold from one individual to the next. Written transcripts of all interview materials were analyzed with this in mind. A schematic representation of the structure used for the data analysis of this study is shown in Figure 1.

The underlying principles of analysis were derived from two axes, the axis of time and the axis of thematic content. Each of these will be discussed in turn.

Pregnancy, as a natural event in the phenomenal world, has a clearly defined beginning (conception) and a clearly defined end (labor and delivery). This in itself was used to sort out the data according to different phases in time and development. The study used the traditional medical practice of dividing pregnancy into three trimesters, but it added three further divisions—conception, labor and delivery, and the postpartum period—to emphasize and separate out specific areas seen as marker events within the overall maternity cycle. Together these six divisions anchored the analysis of the data with reference to time and the natural morphology of pregnancy. They became the basis for the six subsections in chapters 4, 5, and 6.

In addition to the time frame of events occurring during the first pregnancy experience, the pregnancy itself was viewed within the larger time frame of a woman's personal history. Thoughts or issues related to the place and symbolic importance of the pregnancy in each woman's life were thus referred to the larger context of adult development. In this respect the particular structure of the pregnancy as a whole was considered to emerge partially out of life concerns specific to the individual woman and partially from the developmental tasks identified as important for the fourth decade of life.

The second axis of analysis takes up the thematic content of the interviews, a structure derived from the interaction of the minds of the interviewer and the interviewee over time. This structure actually reflects the natural endopsychic structuring of experience by the woman herself

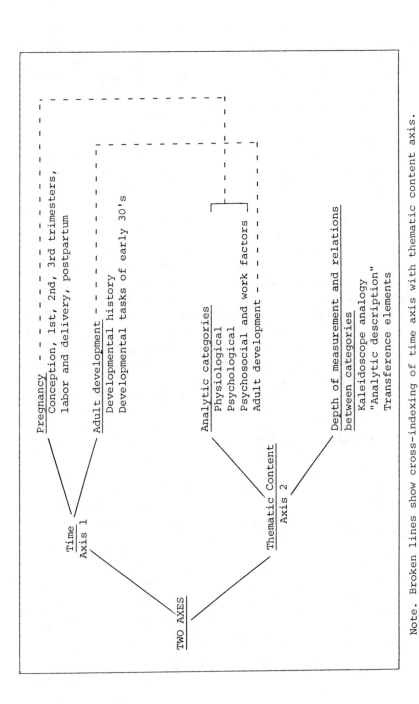

Note. Broken lines show cross-indexing of time axis with thematic content axis.

Figure 1   Structure for Overall Data Analysis

and is therefore one of the major phenomena of the emotional experience of pregnancy. From this perspective, the interviewing process itself becomes a tool for analysis. Shatzman and Strauss (1973) describe this interactive approach as an ongoing "working of thought processes" which begins during data collection and continues through data analysis, leading to what they define as "analytic description." They note:

> a researcher needs to analyze as he goes along both to adjust his observational strategies, shifting some emphases towards those experiences which bear upon the development of his understanding, and generally, to exercise control over his emerging ideas by virtually simultaneous "checking" and "testing" of those ideas. (p. 110)

In this process certain themes or interactions crystallize as significant, while others prove less important.

From the perspective of dynamic psychology, a similar principle is active in the transference (i.e., the exaggerated infantile reactions of psychoanalytic patient to psychoanalyst) which arises out of the therapeutic situation. In this situation, it is the transference which guides the psychoanalyst in his efforts to understand the experiences described. While the interviewing process used in this study did not constitute psychoanalytic psychotherapy, transference elements occasionally emerged, as they do in many other human interactions. Where these occurred, they were included in the data analysis.

At the level of the second axis of analysis, the protocols were thus examined with respect to manifest thematic content and depth of measurement. First, the simpler themes which showed through like beacons in all the protocols were used to establish the main analytic categories: physiological, psychological, psychosocial and work factors, and adult development. The categories are shown in Figure 2 with their further subdivisions into types shown in Figure 3. Next, all the interview material was coded according to the analytic categories. Finally, the coded material in the analytic categories was cross-indexed with reference to the time units making up the first axis of analysis.

At this point, analysis of particular events occurring during a first pregnancy could be approached with the additional aim of devining the relations among different factors as they came together in the overall psychological complex experience of pregnancy. It was these dynamic intermodulating factors which defined the interplay between the woman's experience of herself, of the pregnancy, of her child and her world. This interplay emerged in patterns which could change from week to week, but, as in looking through a kaleidoscope, it was eventually possible to sense certain repeating patterns and, with further familiarity, the orga-

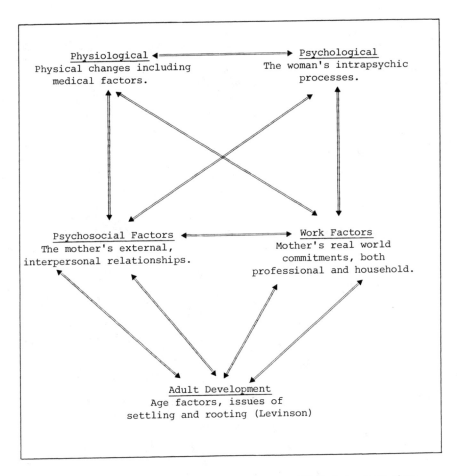

Note. These categories are somewhat artificial in that they imply more separation between the categories than actually exists. The use of this separation is heuristic. The set of categories constitutes an analytic paradigm and serves to allow the data to be more readily understood.

Figure 2   The Categories

Psychological	Self-esteem, self-image factors
	Internal dilemma, conflict or paradox
	Fantasies, dreams, unconscious associations
	Antecedent factors (e.g., previous traumas or pleasures)
	Expectations, mood changes
Physiological	The sleep constellation
	The appetite/digestion constellation
	Illnesses
	The weight constellation
	The energy/fatigue constellation
	Iatrogenic factors (caused by medical intervention) or curative factors
	Medication
Psychosocial	Intercouple factors
	Mother's family of origin factors (past and present)
	Mother's friends
and	Father's family of origin factors (past and present)
	Friends, colleagues
	Reactions from strangers to pregnancy
Work-related Factors	Family responsibilities, the home
	Family responsibilities, outside home
	The work world
Adult Development	Age factors
	Personal history data
	Life structure concepts
	Marker events
	Issues of settling down

Figure 3   The Categories' Subdivisions

nizing principle which defined the interplay of each woman's experience. The kaleidoscope's pattern depends upon:

1. the arrangement of the mirrors;

2. the contents of the kaleidoscope, the shape and color of each individual piece;

3. the interaction of the contents of the kaleidoscope with one another as it is turned;

4. the interaction of the contents of the kaleidoscope with the outside force of gravity.

A similar process of inference and intuition allowed a more comprehensive, in-depth understanding of the experience of pregnancy. By approximate analogy it was possible to consider the four determinants of the kaleidoscope pattern cited above as respectively analogous to:

1. the mother's character structure;

2. the internal experiences of the mother (psychological factors) and their determinants (physical, social, and work factors);

3. the internal dynamic interaction of the mother's psychological factors with one another;

4. the impact of social relations, medical care, the extrinsic physical environment, work relations, with the above.

The effects of pregnancy as an integrating principle in female psychology were thus elaborated with a number of perspectives in mind. This multifaceted approach allowed better understanding of thematic content from different psychological levels. It also facilitated both maximum integration and differentiation of material in any given protocol and across protocols.

The attempt to accommodate the problem of selective extraction from protocols and individual bias was managed by consensual validation of the researcher's concepts through independent collateral examination of the data by one other experienced researcher. Realistically, there is no way to eliminate entirely this type of bias from psychological research. Miller (1969) reports that his experiments on the eyeblink reflex of the rat showed diametrically opposite results in two consecutive four-year periods. He attributed the differences in results to changes in mood of students who were conducting the experiment. Results from the present study are likewise bound by the limitations which attend any examination of natural phenomena. Nevertheless, they may be judged by the same principles which govern any assessment of ordinary experience, namely that the appropriateness of a particular point of view can only be established on the basis that it makes sense in related contexts. From this perspective, the results stand on their merit as a representation of experience with specific explanatory power.

4

Pregnancy: Its Physiological Effects

Results: The Protocols According to the Categories

Results of this study are presented in three separate chapters (4, 5, 6), each with six similar subsections. The three chapters conform to the three categories for analysis described in the methodology: physiological, psychological, and psychosocial. Each chapter is further divided into six subsections reflecting the natural morphology of pregnancy from conception through the three trimesters, to labor and delivery, and the postpartum period. Material from all four protocols will be used to present and illustrate this typology of pregnancy. After this, further analysis in a subsequent chapter will be undertaken to elaborate particular unifying themes and individual characteristics within each protocol. A final chapter will summarize the results obtained with regard to the experience of pregnancy as an integrating principle in female psychology.

Overview

In discussing the physiological effects of pregnancy, it is sometimes difficult to remain consistently within the boundaries of this single category. The tendency to emotionally elaborate physiological experience in life is present during pregnancy as it is generally. Women in this study experienced a range of physical effects during their pregnancies which evoked various emotional and cognitive responses. In the following presentation of the physiological effects of pregnancy, the inevitable interaction of these is reflected by the occasional overlapping of categories.

Conception

All of the women in this study anticipated that conception would be more difficult than it was. In the end, all but one were amazed at how quickly conception occurred. The physical fact of having conceived was closely linked with a positive sense of confirmed fertility as well as a newly implemented dimension of their femininity.

When I skipped a period, I didn't believe I was pregnant at first. I assumed I had skipped a period for other reasons. Then, after 2 weeks, I took in a urine sample. When I was told I was pregnant, I was very surprised at how quickly it had happened. I felt very happy and excited about being fertile. I also felt very proud and womanly and competent and sexy about having been able to do so quickly. (Rachael, conception)

Now that I'm pregnant, I feel like my body's grown up. I feel very womanly. (Katherine, conception)

The one woman who was not suprised by how quickly she became pregnant felt instead that she knew intuitively the moment when she conceived.

So I had in my mind the month I wanted to get pregnant; it just seemed like the right time. And I didn't use birth control this time and I knew when I got pregnant. (Anna, conception)

Her intuitive knowledge, however, did not entirely free her from doubts, because there were no external signs of her pregnancy.

I knew I was pregnant and I was filled with doubts. I don't know—"You don't know you're pregnant; you haven't seen the tests." (Anna, conception)

Only one woman in the study had some trouble conceiving. It turned out later not to be any difficulty with her but rather with her husband. Until the problem was accurately diagnosed, however, this woman went through the very infuriating experience of having her physician propose all kinds of complicated tests to explore her fertility without any suggestion of corresponding investigation for her husband. This example, which occurs as early as conception in this study, reflects a medical obstetrical attitude which typically tends to blame women for difficulties associated with the female reproductive system. The inclination to hold women in some way responsible for their own difficulties, particularly during pregnancy, has been researched by Scully and Bart (1973), who reviewed obstetrical textbooks and discovered that women were generally blamed for a wide range of gynecological and obstetrical problems. Women in this study suffered from this medical bias at various points in their pregnancies when physiological effects were experienced as especially incapacitating or problematic.

The First Trimester

Physical symptoms during pregnancy were most acute in the first and third trimesters. All the women in this study experienced varying degrees of physical symptomatology. Symptoms of the first trimester included generalized fatigue, some feelings of subtle withdrawal from usual preoccupations (perhaps prompted by the increased fatigue) changes in food preferences, and nausea.

All of the women experienced fatigue and feelings of heaviness in their bodies quite early in their pregnancies and were surprised at how quickly these symptoms began to influence their sense of themselves:

> The whole world just seems different. I am amazed at how quickly the pregnancy has changed my existence. I'm real tired. I'm real emotional. Food tastes really different, it is like suddenly I'm on a different planet with food. A lot of things don't taste so good. Coffee, which I usually love, tastes like somebody put a tire in hot water and burned rubber. Everything just seems like a lot of work. I just feel physically real exhausted from it. That was kind of a shock. I guess I expected to feel that way at the end of pregnancy and not at the beginning. (Rachael, 10 weeks)

> So during these early weeks of pregnancy, I haven't had physical illness at all, except sometimes I've felt tired. I've sometimes felt like a junkie nodding off in a bus. The body changes are so subtle. My metabolism reacts so supersensitively to caffeine and alcohol, I've completely lost my taste for both. (Anna, 9 weeks)

Another prevalent symptom of pregnancy—nausea—was experienced by all but one of the women in the study. Of the three women who experienced nausea, two experienced a moderate amount of it which tapered off by the end of the first trimester, while one found her entire experience of the first trimester dominated by this single symptom.

Described as "morning sickness," nausea during pregnancy can actually occur at any time of day or throughout the day, every day. In relation to pregnancy, nausea has been the object of much theorizing and speculation from both psychoanalytic and medical points of view. Despite the fact that nausea and vomiting are commonly believed to be aggravated by psychological factors, research evidence regarding this assumption is inconclusive and contradictory (Sherman, 1971). There is little agreement in the literature about which biological, psychological, or sociological factors are associated with this symptom, nor is it known what proportion of pregnant women actually experience it (Trethowan & Dickens, 1972). It is known that biochemical changes occurring in pregnancy result in a lowered threshold for vomiting. Grimm (1967) concludes from this that nausea and vomiting in pregnancy are not necessarily signs of maladjustment or rejection of the pregnancy. The psychoanalytic understanding of nausea during pregnancy, however, believes otherwise, consistently linking this symptom to psychogenic factors. The intensity and duration of nausea is seen as a reflection of a woman's unconscious feelings about her pregnancy and, by extension, her child (Chertok, 1969). The difficulty with this line of reasoning is that, in accord with it, making conscious this unconscious rejection of the pregnancy should naturally result in some symptomatic relief.

That such a result is not always forthcoming is illustrated by one of the women in this study. Linda experienced extreme nausea almost continuously throughout her pregnancy. She was also quite able to articulate her ambivalence and even hatred of what was happening to her. Yet her nausea continued, abating only slightly after the first trimester.

> I was sick like most women are, I guess, at first. I was nauseous all the time; and then it got to the point where I've been throwing up all the time. And I'm either throwing up or so nauseous that I cannot do anything. Nothing helps. I call Birthways every day and cry on the phone and say, "What can I do?" and they say, "Take B vitamins," and nothing, nothing, nothing works. (Linda, 9 weeks)

Linda was aware of the psychoanalytic position that nausea during pregnancy is tied to unconscious feelings about the child. Her awareness of this theoretical position increased her confusion over the severity of her physical condition and came to affect her self-image throughout her pregnancy in negative ways.

> I feel sort of like that the attitude I am getting from people—and also that I believe inside myself—is that I am sick because of my ambivalence and if I could only get it together and decide, "Look, this is what you're doing with your life now, just give it up and don't be ambivalent," that I would not be sick any more. And I feel like there probably is some truth to the fact that I am having emotional ambivalence, but I mean, what's the cause and what's the effect? I feel a lot like the ambivalence is because I am so damned sick. (Linda, 9 weeks)

The intensity of her physical response to pregnancy in the first trimester was totally unanticipated. She had never imagined she could be so sick from being pregnant. In fact, she had thought she might enjoy her pregnancy. She was 35 years old when she conceived, had looked forward to having a child, and was settled in a secure marital relationship. As her life came to be completely dominated by her nausea in these first four months, she experienced real conflict over being pregnant and even considered the possibility of ending the pregnancy. She ultimately decided she would continue her pregnancy, but continued to find her sense of herself impaired by her physical symptoms.

The other women in the study experienced milder forms of nausea and generally less discomfort in early pregnancy. Interestingly enough, the woman who had the least number of symptoms also had the most difficulty convincing her husband that she was pregnant. Her husband kept saying that she seemed too well to be pregnant.

And even after I had the [pregnancy] test, I didn't have any physical symptoms; I felt great. He couldn't see anything, and I wasn't sick, and he just was filled with real anxiety that I was not really pregnant. (Anna, 5 weeks)

Between these two extremes of physical response to pregnancy, there may be an optimum level of symptomatology in early pregnancy which sets in motion a process of initial attachment to the pregnancy. It is clear that, if the physical symptoms are too severe, there is a negative effect on the woman's self-image, her relationship with the pregnancy becomes conflicted, and a real psychological problem develops. If there is little or no physical symptomatology, on the other hand, the pregnancy may rest primarily on internal conviction. The appearance of physical symptoms commonly associated with pregnancy—fatigue, discomfort, heaviness, and nausea—first made these women aware that the actual experience of having a child was unpredictable in its physical course. In this way, the physical experience was different than the imagination of it had been prior to conception. Prior to conception, these women had had a growing sense of wanting a child. That idea had become more and more distinct until it was carried into reality through conception. With the initiation of that physical experience and the subsequent first trimester came the first reality of the idea or fantasy of having a child. The first part of pregnancy, with its initial array of physical symptoms, appears to function primarily as a period of gradual reorientation from external to internal awareness. Physical symptoms at this time seem to help a woman connect to her pregnancy in a concrete, generally positive way, as long as the symptoms are not overwhelming.

Less common physical symptoms appear to trigger fantasies more related to the potential for difficulty with the pregnancy. Two of the women in this study had the experience of temporary symptoms which were difficult to explain. Both women immediately associated them with possible complications with the pregnancy. Rachael, who had blood in her urine, wondered if she might be growing a tumor along with the child.

I had some physical problems at the beginning and I was concerned that I might have either a problem with my kidneys or a tumor or something going on in my body at the same time as I was pregnant. (Rachael, 11 weeks)

Anna, who experienced a sudden pain in her abdomen which lasted for about an hour, immediately wondered about the possibility of a tubal pregnancy or an "abnormal pregnant state." The content of their distressful fantasies was closely aligned to the stage of embryonic development in the first trimester. In these months, the fetus is at its most vulnerable and the viability of the pregnancy is still in question. Fortunately, the temporary nature of their symptoms eventually allowed these women to be reassured about their condition.

Out of the experience of conception and the first months of pregnancy, women in this study also began to develop a different perspective about their bodies. Apart from Anna, who knew intuitively when she conceived, the other three women were surprised at the speed of conception as though they hadn't quite believed that their bodies would respond so reliably in this quintessentially feminine way. After conception, apart from various physical symptoms, changes in the body, such as increased breast size and an unaccustomed roundness in the belly, were viewed positively.

> I am basically feeling a little bit rounder and kind of liking that roundness. It feels cuddly or something like that. (Rachael, 11 weeks)

These feelings shifted as the pregnancy progressed. Their development will be presented in the next sections.

Overall, the extent of physical symptomatology in the early months of pregnancy varies considerably from woman to woman. Despite individual differences, however, women found that the reality of pregnancy tended to be validated by the presence of physical symptoms. It is one of the ways a woman is certain she is really carrying a child. The reality she feels in this way is also more easily communicated to her husband. Besides affirming the reality of pregnancy, physical symptoms require a woman to pay more attention to herself, thus initiating the beginnings of more specific maternal feeling. Mothering behavior and maternal feeling are not unfamiliar to women who may have exhibited such behavior or experienced such feelings in childhood play with dolls or perhaps in caring for other children. But the sense of being a mother—oneself—to a specific child—one's own—is first developed during pregnancy. Even women who spoke of having "always liked children" found themselves feeling somewhat surprisingly *unmotherly* when it came to maternal feelings in relation to their own fetus during the first trimester. The development of maternal feeling is in part aligned with the physical changes which occur throughout pregnancy. By requiring a woman to pay more attention to her physical self, symptoms stimulate bodily preoccupation, drawing a woman's attention to her unborn child—who is, for the moment, primarily experienced as a physical discomfort in the form of fatigue, nausea, or other symptoms.

The Second Trimester

The main physical events of the second trimester are the quickening*
when fetal movements first appear, and the increasing size of the body so
that by the end of the second trimester women look visibly pregnant. The
second trimester also brings a decrease in symptoms such as nausea and
women generally feel better physically, although shortness of breath, increased frequency of urination, and concern with weight become issues
at this time.

By the end of the first trimester and moving into the second, all the
women in this study began to notice more roundness in the abdomen and
increased breast size. These changes were first viewed as positive. Katherine, at four months, was excited about the way she looked:

> This is the first week my belly felt big! My body looks pregnant, and it's exciting.
> (Katherine, 16 weeks)

But these initial feelings of pleasure in the physical roundness of
pregnancy soon began to alternate with less pleasurable feelings as the
second trimester continued. Fears about their attractiveness as women
began to surface as their bodies expanded. Rachael, who felt very positively about her body at four months, found herself beginning to worry
about her weight only one month later.

> I'm struggling with my body image. I've always had to worry about being plump and
> I feel cumbersome now, so I wonder about feeding the baby versus gaining weight.
> (Rachael, 20 weeks)

It became important to be perceived as attractively pregnant rather
than simply fat. Anna experienced discomfort with her appearance early
in the second trimester just before quickening.

> My body is changing. I feel like I don't look pregnant. I may be perceived as getting
> fat by others. I don't like that. My breasts are bigger and my belly, too. I feel uncom-
> fortable about the way that I look. (Anna, 16 weeks)

Even Katherine, who felt so positively about "looking pregnant" at four
months, found her body image beginning to fluctuate in its appeal by the
fifth month and felt ambivalent about her appearance.

*Quickening: feeling fetal movements for the first time. (Taken from *Birth of a First
Child*, Breen, 1975.)

Sometimes I feel big and awkward, like I need to waddle. Other times it feels like I am trim, vital, and vigorous. When I feel big, I don't like it. It makes me feel like there is an appendage I can't get accustomed to. (Katherine, 21 weeks)

For Linda, who had experienced special difficulties in the first trimester, the sense of getting larger was overshadowed in the early weeks of the second trimester by the hope that the end of the first trimester would bring some relief from the nausea. This did not immediately occur. The disappointment that things did not improve as much as she hoped left Linda feeling uncertain about the changes in her body.

I've been living day by day at this point. I've just been surviving. I'm not sure how I feel about the pregnancy. I've been sort of in shock from what it's been like. (Linda, 17 weeks)

Lessened satisfaction with their bodies, however, was somewhat off-set at this time by the event of quickening. Women felt the baby's first movements at slightly different times between 18 and 21 weeks. The quickening affected all the women profoundly and inaugurated a new phase in their relationship with the fetus. There was now a vivid sense of being two in this pregnancy: themselves and an infant who was definitely more separate from them. The quickening was an important confirmation of an already-felt sense of carrying a living being. From then on, the fetal movements became a means of more direct communication between mother and unborn child. While the movement initially felt odd to one woman due to the novelty of the experience, it remained a highly valued indication of the liveness of the fetus once she grew accustomed to it.

The baby started moving. It feels a little like falling. I'm sort of scared of it. The only thing I've experienced quite like that before was stomach distress or my heart beating fast, or something that meant things are not okay. (18 weeks) . . . then I realized I was attached to the movement when a day went by when the baby didn't move and I really missed it. (Rachael, 19 weeks)

Attachment to the fetal movements was felt by all the women. Each of them learned to distinguish between different types of movements and experienced them as a form of communication with their child. Pleasure in these movements was at its height in the second trimester. The close association between carrying a child and gaining weight was reinforced by these movements and helped to cushion some of the negative feelings women progressively experienced about their bodies. Anna, who felt uncomfortable with her appearance at four months, worried more about her increased appetite and weight just before she felt her baby move. Once the baby moved, she felt better about her body and her appetite. Concern for her baby's health also changed Katherine's feelings about her food intake during the second trimester.

> I'm 25 pounds over what I ordinarily am, but my feelings are totally different now about my weight. I want a big baby because birth weight is linked to basic health later in life. I am concerned about nutrition. Before, when I was alone in my body, I would binge and then diet. Now I can't do that. (Katherine, 22 weeks)

At the same time, the changes in her physical size made Katherine wonder how her body was adjusting to the added strains of pregnancy.

> I've had uncomfortable pulling sensations in my body lately. It raises fears about how my body is faring in pregnancy. (Katherine, 21 weeks)

Thus, physical changes in the second trimester which are initially viewed as pleasurable and positive became more conflicted as the boundary line between being perceived as "fat" and being perceived as pregnant was reached. This growing visibility of the pregnancy, as well as the quickening which established a vivid sense of an internal "other," became events that moved a woman from the private, even secret, world of the first trimester, where the choice of sharing her pregnancy with others still remained, to the more complex and differentiated sphere of public interaction with a wider set of social and work relations. Again, these changes were coupled with feelings of ambivalence. Katherine expressed both sides of the ambivalence clearly, feeling alternately pleased and upset:

> Other people are beginning to notice. They are interested in a really nice way. I talk about it more eagerly, too. I feel more legitimate now in the second trimester. (Katherine, 17 weeks)

> I've been distressed this week. I'm anxious about being so visibly pregnant. I'm too large to ignore and other people are noticing. All these months I've wanted to look more pregnant, now it's so visible. (Katherine, 20 weeks)

Despite increasing ambivalence about the physical changes of pregnancy, women in this study generally enjoyed their pregnancies most in the second trimester. Fewer symptoms, the fetal movements, and increased attention from their environment combined to make these months more satisfying than the other trimesters.

The Third Trimester

The third trimester was characterized by an increase in physical symptoms and overall discomfort, with increased negativity toward the physical appearance of late pregnancy. There was also anxiety directed toward the impending labor and delivery. All the women in the study started birth classes in the third trimester, further emphasizing the imminence of labor and delivery.

Physical symptoms of the third trimester included restlessness, insomnia, some return of nausea, feelings of fatigue at times alternating with bursts of energy, swelling of feet, and water retention. There was also at this time a greater preoccupation with the external world in terms of making active preparations for the baby's room, clothes, and toys. The real physical discomfort with the pregnancy in this trimester appeared to play an important part in preparing a woman to separate from her child at childbirth. It was the physical discomfort which, above all, made women eager to have the pregnancy end. Whereas physical symptoms in the first trimester helped to establish the reality of pregnancy, physical symptoms in the third trimester stimulated impatience with the pregnancy and a desire for it to end.

> I'm more physically uncomfortable. Ligaments on the insides of my legs are sore. The muscle knots in my back and below my breasts. I'm tired and feel ready not to be pregnant any more. I want to have this baby and have it be over with. I want my body back. (Rachael, 27 weeks)

Continued growth of the abdomen left women in this study feeling big and cumbersome in the third trimester, increasing their sense of frustration with the pregnancy.

> I'm feeling very pregnant, very big. I feel like a walrus, big and lumbering. I have to roll over to sit up. I get frustrated that I can't move so fast. (Katherine, 28 weeks)

> Taking a shower has been a real endeavor, because I can't get my arms over my belly. (Linda, 29 weeks)

Even the fetal movements, highly valued as they were and continued to be, came to be viewed with more ambivalence at this time. The sense that the baby was not only separate from the self, but at times an intrusion on the self, was reinforced by the increased physical discomfort associated with its movements in the womb.

> The baby's kicking a lot more. It's fun when I lay back and think about this. Yet I feel so much that it's a foreign body. I had thought I would feel more connected, more oneness with the baby, but it feels like this is a separate being. I get irritated when the baby kicks me and it hurts. (Katherine, 28 weeks)

> I don't always like the movement now. It's become increasingly intrusive in my life, uncomfortable and painful. I feel like I'm getting bruised ribs and a squished-up stomach. (Rachael, 30 weeks)

Feelings of disorientation and poor coordination appeared in the weeks just before childbirth. At times this was coupled with new feelings of disconnection from the child.

> The baby is not moving so much. It is getting more indistinct, like it's gone into a fog . . . I have very poor coordination and I'm getting forgetful. Somehow I'm not paying attention to where I'm going. (Rachael, 35 weeks)

> I'm getting up at night. I can't sleep and get disoriented. So I get up to see what time it is. (Katherine, 32 weeks)

> I am focused on the delivery. I'm feeling resistant to being with the baby. (Anna, 34 weeks)

More and more, attention shifted to the prospect of childbirth and the anticipated pleasure of finally holding a child of one's own. It was also at this time that one of the women found out she would be giving birth by Caesarean section due to her baby's position in the womb and the size of the baby's head. This discovery evoked a grief reaction at first but was eventually accepted as a necessity for the added safety of the delivery. In this way, the last weeks of pregnancy were spent in mental and physical preparation for the labor and delivery, which all the women regarded with genuine apprehension in terms of the ordeal it represented.

Overall, the bodily changes experienced by these women during pregnancy were accompanied by a variety of physical symptoms and evoked a range of ambivalent feelings. While feelings of pleasure about appearing pregnant and developing a more mature figure existed, the physical changes of pregnancy proved increasingly difficult to adapt to and, not surprisingly, women tended to view their bodies as vulnerable throughout this entire period. It is a striking characteristic of pregnancy that it is the only period in adult life during which major bodily changes occur with great rapidity and under normal circumstances.

To what extent feelings about the physical changes were influenced by cultural values as well as subjective perceptions of simple discomfort was difficult to determine. It is true that pregnancy is not free from physical discomfort. It is also true that being pregnant in a culture which conditions women to derive much of their self-worth from their appearance, and which highly values a slender appearance, is likely to influence the way a woman feels about her increased size and weight. While pregnant women are often depicted as looking especially radiant, women themselves feel more ambivalent about their looks and this ambivalence increases as pregnancy continues. Women also express ambivalence about the physiological effects of pregnancy. While initial symptoms may be accepted as a confirmation of the pregnancy, ongoing physical discomfort gives rise to the desire for the pregnancy to end so a more normal sense of self may be reclaimed.

Labor and Delivery

All four women in this study had attended childbirth classes in the last months of pregnancy and were planning a natural childbirth in an alternative birth center or, in Katherine's case, at home. Of the four women, three had long labors, one of them ending in an unplanned Caesarean section. One woman, who discovered just a few weeks before her due date that she would have to have a Caesarean section, had the operation shortly after labor began.

All of the women experienced labor and delivery as a period of intense physical challenge. They found themselves amazed at the amount of pain experienced and exhausted by the length of labor.

> It was a much more powerful experience than I think I was prepared for, and a much more painful experience than I think I was prepared for. I think I had ingested some of the romantic notions of natural childbirth that if you just breathed right, it wasn't gonna hurt. And there was no way it wasn't gonna hurt! Or wasn't gonna hurt more than anything had ever hurt me in my life. And that was something of a shock to experience and a shock to have to experience for so long. (Rachael, labor and delivery)

At the same time, the excitement of at last delivering a baby and seeing their child buffered the level of physical distress for these women. Linda, whose baby was delivered by C-section, reacted with an excitement typical of all the women.

> And my husband took my head and turned it around so that we would be looking at each other, while we heard the baby cry. And we were both crying. And that was the third most wonderful moment of my whole life. (Linda, labor and delivery)

Once the baby was born, even though Linda's physical ordeal was not over as her doctor proceeded to give her medicine she was allergic to, she found that her attention was more focused on the excitement of delivery than anything else.

> Meanwhile, they were sewing me up and that took about another 45 minutes; and then I was in the delivery room, throwing up [laughs]. Talk about the pattern of my pregnancy—But they had given me demerol and I was allergic to demerol, so I threw up about 16 times. But it was no big deal. I mean, God, it was just so anticlimactic. (Linda, labor and delivery)

For Anna and Katherine, who both delivered vaginally, there was the added satisfaction of having had a childbirth closer to what they had originally wanted. Linda and Rachael, on the other hand, had to overcome their disappointment at delivering their babies by Caesarean section. Linda, who had been forewarned about the intended operation, worked through her disappointment in advance. She was able to accept her situation and responded to the actual delivery with great excitement. Rachael worked through her feelings of disappointment more in retrospect. At the time the decision was made, she was so exhausted and concerned about the baby's safety that she experienced only gratitude and relief that it would soon be over. The sense of disappointment came later for her.

> I was prepared for a natural childbirth and then, although I went into labor around my due date, wound up in labor for about 48 hours and eventually when my uterus began to close again, rather than dilating further, the doctors, my husband, and I made the decision to go ahead and have a Caesarean since there was really no other way around it at that point. So I wound up with a C-section and a stay in the hospital, which wasn't planned and certainly a more medical delivery than I hoped for, planning to deliver in an alternative birth center with no drugs and all that kind of thing. So it was very much of a shock. And it was a very overwhelming and terrible experience in a lot of ways. About the labor, I felt real disappointed; I felt at the same time that I have no regrets about how I handled it . . . (Rachael, labor and delivery)

Anna, though she delivered vaginally, also needed medical intervention. After her contractions began and then subsided again, she was given medication to strengthen the contractions, making them more powerful and closer together. She also experienced labor as physically more challenging than she had anticipated.

> They were very rapid and the contractions were very close together and strong from the beginning . . . and I was quite awed by the power. I mean I was just awed by the power involved in it. After a while, it sort of just gets beyond pain. (Anna, labor and delivery)

Approximately 28 hours after labor began, the doctor decided to use forceps to deliver. Like Rachael, Anna accepted the decision with relief. The physical sensation, however, was quite overwhelming and led to a moment of panic when she could no longer hear the baby's heartbeat on the fetal monitor due to her changed position. Like the other women, once the baby was born, Anna found her attention focused only on her child. This shift in attention began during the final part of labor and continued after delivery.

> I couldn't have cared where he was born. I had put a lot of emphasis on A.B.C. [Alternative Birth Center]. . . . But frankly, it didn't matter to me where he was born. I had no awareness beyond probably a perimeter of two feet on either side of me. I didn't care where I was. It had nothing to do with me. Whether I was delivering in the

A.B.C. or this sterile delivery room, it just didn't matter. But that's something probably you don't think about when you're early in labor. You're more focused on your surroundings. . . . During the end of labor, it was like I had tunnel vision, really tunnel vision. I have returned to that labor room and floor since the birth. The first few times I was there, I could swear to you that that wasn't the place I was. It doesn't look the same. It just was a totally different visual perception of where I was. (Anna, labor and delivery)

In keeping with new trends in medical obstetrics, which are beginning to show some response to growing demands from the women's movement, and new research demonstrating the importance of minimizing medical intervention during the birth process, women in this study remained awake during delivery and were allowed to hold their infants immediately after childbirth. Nonetheless, all but Katherine, who delivered at home, were separated from their infants for brief periods after the birth for various reasons. Linda and Rachael, who were themselves suffering from the surgical intervention of a C-section, responded somewhat less intensely to the experience of momentary separation from their infants, but Anna found even the briefest separation painful. She experienced the separation as a traumatic disruption of the exceedingly delicate bonding process she had begun with her child upon first holding him.

I felt deprived about my first moments with my son. They were cut off too soon. I could have spent hours feeling the feelings of connectedness with him just after he was born. Instead they took him from me to move us into another room. We were together again immediately, but the "moment" was definitely interrupted. (Anna, labor and delivery)

For all of these women, labor and delivery proved to be a dramatic and critical period of transition drawing on all of their physical and emotional reserves. For each woman, the physical experience of childbirth was an ordeal of significantly greater proportions than they had anticipated. Each woman also found some measure of her self-esteem attached to the way she handled the physical stress and pain involved. Rachael and Anna felt that they had done their best and came away from the experience feeling strong about themselves. Linda, who had experienced an unusually difficult pregnancy, found the delivery at first yet another disappointment because it denied her the experience of testing herself in labor as she had looked forward to. Katherine, who delivered at home without medical intervention or anesthesia, felt satisfied with her experience except for one moment when she felt herself crumbling in the face of the intense pain she was experiencing. At that point she realized that, had she been in a hospital, she would have asked for anesthesia. The realization came as a surprise. She had anticipated that her natural childbirth training would have prevented her from experiencing what she perceived as a loss of emotional control. Other than this, she was pleased to have delivered at home in familiar surroundings in the presence of close friends and with the help of a midwife.

Clearly, retaining some sense of mastery of their situation appeared important for these women in their response to childbirth as a difficult, painful, though ultimately rewarding event. In addition, the physical presence of their newborn and the opportunity to immediately see and hold the child acted as a partial buffer to further pain and discomfort after delivery.

Postpartum

The early postpartum weeks were a period of delicate physical and emotional adjustment between mother and child. For the mother they were also a period of readjustment to no longer being pregnant. During the first six weeks after childbirth, called the puerperium, the most rapid changes returning the body to its nonpregnant state normally occur. Lactation and nursing aid in this process, both by stimulating uterine contractions and by temporarily inhibiting ovulation and menstruation, thus ensuring that no new pregnancy will occur.

All of the women in this study decided early in pregnancy to breast-feed their babies. Two women experienced no particular difficulty in establishing nursing, while two experienced some initial difficulty, but overcame these problems and eventually nursed their infants successfully. All the women found the nursing relationship a richly rewarding experience, although it did tie them down more than would otherwise have been the case.

Fatigue and concern over permanent body changes as a result of pregnancy were also voiced by these women postpartum. Fatigue and lack of sleep were particularly prominent in the early weeks of postpartum and continued for much longer than the women had expected.

> I also didn't know that a person could be as fatigued as I was. I didn't know that kind of exhaustion existed in the world, and I was overwhelmed by my exhaustion. I didn't know what a powerful impact a physical feeling can have on you. It went on probably for 6 months. I started to feel more energy around 5 months, but I was very, very tired for the first 3 months. That seemed overwhelming to me at times. "How do I repair this physical rip in my make-up? How do I make my energy come back?" I used to ask myself. (Anna, postpartum)

Part of the dilemma, postpartum, as far as the fatigue was concerned, was the mother's need for rest necessarily conflicting with the realities of infant care.

Taking care of a baby is more work than I ever did about anything. I remember early on, after she was born, I used to think constantly about people like vice-presidents in charge of GM or something, and I used to think, I dare you to come into my house and try to do what I'm doing. I used to think about that all the time, because I have never in my life done so much work as I have done with a baby. And, of course, you're not prepared for that either. (Linda, postpartum)

The sense of having a different body as a result of the pregnancy was felt to various degrees. Rachael felt physically more vulnerable after having had a C-section, particularly when she thought of having another child. Linda, who had had a large baby, felt quite negatively about the changes in her body.

Because my baby was 10-6½ at birth, I had an enormous stomach and I stretched totally out of shape; and I have lots and lots of stretch marks—and don't like that at all and feel like my body will never be the same. (Linda, postpartum)

The increased sense of physical vulnerability at times extended to the renewal of sexual relations with the husband. Katherine felt this especially vividly.

I realized I was scared to have sex. I had fantastic images of being hurt, ramrodded. It was very much connected with the pain of delivery. (Katherine, postpartum)

Summary

This portrayal of the physiological effects of a first pregnancy as experienced by these women is in contrast to popular views of pregnancy as an illness or as a passive period of more or less self-indulgent withdrawal. It appears that pregnancy brings with it physical changes and accommodations which are characteristically perceived with increasing ambivalence by all the women as pregnancy progresses. To what extent the physical process of pregnancy activates and interacts with important psychological processes that facilitate the developing sense of relatedness with the baby, the evolution of maternal feeling, and the incorporation of the baby within the marriage are the subjects of the next chapters.

5

Pregnancy: Its Psychological Effects

Overview

The physiological aspects of maternity, from conception on through all the stages of the reproductive cycle including development of relations with the newborn child, remain more directly observable than their psychological counterparts. Popular stereotypes of the pregnant woman depict her as blissfully withdrawn and dreamy, as emotionally less stable and at times even rather childish in her sudden cravings or dislikes for particular foods. The experience of women in this study partially supports some of these more popular views, but, as is often the case with stereotypes, also diverges from them to reveal a considerably more complex portrait of the psychological effects of pregnancy.

Conception

A striking finding of this study is the extent to which all the women in the study were emotionally preoccupied with the prospect of becoming pregnant long before pregnancy actually occurred. To what extent this preoccupation is a reflection of these women's earlier choice to delay childbearing, and to what extent it is a reflection of their maturity and the realistic anticipation that having a child would be likely to have a profound impact on their relationships with their husbands are uncertain. The fact remains that all of these women spent from several months to a year and a half thinking about their desire to have a child and evaluating their life situation in terms of its readiness to incorporate a child. Without exception, the stability and depth of the marital relationship were determining factors in finally deciding to conceive a child. Rachael, for example, while somewhat concerned about the biological aspects of age (she was 31 when she conceived and hoped eventually to have a second child to complete her family), felt that her desire to have a child could only be fulfilled when her relationship with her husband became thoroughly comfortable.

> James and I lived together 4 and ½ years. We started to feel very secure with each other, and with that, the desire for a baby grew. When we decided to go ahead and have a baby, we talked about marriage. We started trying to have a baby about 1 week before we got married and the baby was probably conceived around then. (Rachael, conception)

Katherine and Linda also felt this combination of factors—the need for marital stability and the biological pressure of being in their 30s. Yet, for each of them, the marital relationship remained the more important determining factor. Anna, who felt an unusual connection with her child even prior to conception, spent a year and a half after having decided to have a child preparing herself and her relationship with her husband to the point where she felt ready to conceive.

> There was a night about a year and a half before I got pregnant when I was looking at the full moon, standing on that little bedroom deck. And looking up at the moon, I felt this strong beam of—a feeling of love; and how I interpreted that was that this was a being who wanted to come through me. And at that time I made an agreement with that—I'll call it a being, that I would bring myself—do the work I felt I needed to do, to bring myself to this point where I felt I would be ready to actually get pregnant. I felt like I needed to do a lot of internal work and mostly it involved my relationship with John, really bringing that to the fore and shining my light on that relationship, me in that relationship. (Anna, conception)

Thus, conception itself was closely linked, for these women, to an emotional evaluation of the marital relationship and a sense of personal readiness to take on the responsibilities of motherhood.

Once the decision to conceive was made, women found that making love with the intent to conceive a child could add a special dimension to the intimacy of sexual intercourse.

> Making love to get pregnant made me feel special, more cosmic, like there were basically these male and female things—like dipping into this undercurrent of life and producing new life. (Rachael, conception)

At the same time, continuing efforts could also make the woman feel somewhat mechanical as she concentrated on getting pregnant as soon as possible after making the decision to have a child.

> It took us 2 months to get pregnant, and by the second month, I was sort of feeling like it was—I felt a little bit like a robot, doing the sex-determining because we decided we wanted a girl. (Linda, conception)

In each case, confirmation of having conceived was considered an exciting event leading to an enhanced sense of adult femininity and personal commitment to the marital relationship.

I couldn't have a baby if I didn't feel completely committed to the man involved. My relationship with John, how open it is and how committed I am, was in direct correlation to my willingness to get pregnant. They existed completely parallel-ly for me. (Anna, conception)

Having a baby made me feel finally like an adult. My body will finally become a woman's body. (Katherine, conception)

For these women, the decision to conceive and become pregnant was tied to careful personal evaluation and deep interpersonal commitment. Within this positive emotional framework, however, the psychological effects of pregnancy were nonetheless distressing and at times disorienting, demonstrating that some of the turmoil of pregnancy is normal and may indeed be linked to the developmental task of making the transition to motherhood.

The First Trimester

Many of the emotional changes during pregnancy have been explained as peripheral, symptomatic effects of the vastly changed hormonal balance which is a part of pregnancy. While changes in hormonal patterns definitely exist, sole reliance on physiological explanations for the emotional aspects of pregnancy denies women the significance of their feelings and avoids understanding the psychological and social factors that help shape a woman's experience of pregnancy. It also fails to take into account the reality that gestating another person inside one's body is bound to have emotional significance far beyond any other normal physical state. In fact, women in this study very early in pregnancy felt themselves to be emotionally different as a result of being pregnant. These differences continued to be amplified throughout pregnancy, labor, delivery, and postpartum.

The first trimester forms a woman's initial adjustment to pregnancy. All of the women in this study reported mood changes. Mild depression, increased emotional sensitivity, and a new sense of separateness from others who were not pregnant emerged.

And my husband didn't have that inner sense of trust that I felt [about the pregnancy], because he wasn't in me. And that was the beginning of this theme about the pregnancy of "Nobody's sharing this with me; nobody knows this or feels the things I feel, and I can't make somebody feel what I feel." That has been painful. I think the first couple of months this has been a real recurring theme, of being totally separate and alone and lonely, just lonely. (Anna, 8 weeks)

I feel real alone about being pregnant. People give me lots of advice but don't listen. (Katherine, 10 weeks)

Some of these feelings of separateness or aloneness in the pregnancy experience seemed to be a part of a shifting psychological orientation.

Even in the earliest weeks of pregnancy, long before the pregnancy was visible to any outsider, the women began to sense themselves becoming less available to the usual concerns of their world. A slight dizziness, a moment of absentmindedness, a passing disinterest in a normally interesting conversation with a friend were often the earliest manifestations of this gradual shift in psychological focus. In these ways, women began to sense themselves to be not quite themselves. The sleepiness and mood alteration of early pregnancy came to reflect this shift for Anna. They drew her away from others and took her deeper within herself as a result of the newly begun life within her.

> I am feeling fatigue often. Sometimes I experience feeling depressed. Two weeks ago I was feeling depressed and felt fearful about exploring or allowing the depression. When I let it happen, my feeling was of wanting to withdraw into myself and what I found there I still experience when this feeling comes up, is a vast wilderness. I experience myself as a miniature, very tiny yet visually a perfect image of myself . . . When I am within myself, it's such an effort to come out, as though language is too difficult and coming "outside" again too far away and such a long journey. (Anna, 5 weeks)

The sense of separateness, of being alone in the experience of her pregnancy remained an important theme for Anna. The same was true for Linda, although she expressed it differently. The feeling of aloneness and isolation were greatly aggravated for her because she spent the first trimester so shocked and overwhelmed by the extent of her physical illness as a result of pregnancy.

> I feel sick and tired much of the time. I have difficulty eating, so my husband and I don't share meals together. It makes me sick to see what he is eating. I just feel overwhelmed by it. I feel isolated from Tim and from the world. (Linda, 7 weeks)

Her sense of isolation was deepened by her surprise that pregnancy could be so physically debilitating. Her images of pregnancy had been typical of the blissful, dreamy stereotypes. Now her anger and resentment emerged in the form of, "Why is this happening to me and why didn't anyone tell me pregnancy would be this way?" Believing that pregnancy should be easy for a woman, her sense of self began to suffer as her own experience continued to diverge from her image of what was supposed to happen and how she was supposed to feel.

> I feel bad about myself. Some of it has to do with just being a woman. If you're a real woman, then having a baby is like rolling off a log. Women just have babies, right? And it's not that way at all for me. (Linda, 9 weeks)

Rachael and Katherine, who also experienced feelings of separateness as a result of being pregnant, felt the separateness more in terms of a heightened emotional sensitivity. Feelings of depression, teariness, and vulnerability contributed to making "the whole world seem different."

At the same time, somewhat paradoxically perhaps (unless one remembers that pregnancy differs from all other physical conditions because it involves the gestation of a person) women felt pleased about being pregnant and expressed feelings of well-being in spite of the increased physical and emotional distress of the first trimester.

> And still there is the disbelief and the joy and the awe that I really am pregnant and there really is going to be a baby. (Rachael, 10 weeks)

The sense of being isolated and alone, as well as physically stressed because of being pregnant, was coupled with a feeling of purpose in having a child. The tasks of pregnancy are not simply biological. They involve the gradual emergence of the woman's psychological sense of her child as a separate locus of feelings, motivations, and intentions which are experienced in increasingly human terms.

Beginning in the first trimester, all the women in this study noted an intensification of their fantasy life and their dreams. It is likely that, as these women felt themselves more separate from others and became more introspective, they simultaneously became more aware of their inner life and so were naturally carried deeper into their subjective fantasies. They also reported an increase in the number of dreams with themes related to pregnancy and motherhood. This is in keeping with findings from an earlier study on the manifest content of dreams of pregnant women (Gillman, 1968). When pregnant women were compared with nonpregnant women of the same age, this study found that approximately 40% of the dreams of pregnant women were about having a baby, as opposed to 1% of the dreams of nonpregnant women. Dreams in the first trimester brought up associations to the pregnancy emphasizing expanding fertility and themes of transformation. Anna began having dreams she associated with pregnancy in the first weeks after conception.

> I've had several dreams that I've associated with pregnancy. One of them was being in a landscape like Yellowstone Park, which is filled with thermal features. My parents, brother, John, and I are going through somebody's cottage, looking through the cupboards and I find branchwater in the cupboard. I notice that the living room furniture is my furniture, arranged just like a normal living room around these three steam beds that were coming deep out of the ground. (Anna, 5 weeks)

For her, the thermal features and the sense of "all this activity underground" were associated with being pregnant. Katherine also had dreams in the early weeks of pregnancy that she associated with becoming more feminine because she was pregnant.

> I was in a fashion show. The blouse I was wearing had become a silky, glamorous, ruffled blouse. I was previously wearing a simple, white cotton Indian blouse. I was now trying on a series of skirts rather than trousers. (Katherine, 5 weeks)

Apprehension and anxiety about pregnancy were also present in dreams. Katherine, when she found herself without a lady's slip in her "fashion show" dream, wondered if she had "all the necessary equipment to be a female." Linda, who felt to some extent trapped by her physical distress in pregnancy, dreamed of being caught in a long tunnel from which she could not escape. She found the dream very frightening. It symbolized for her the sense of being caught in a process from which there was no escape except through childbirth which she also feared.

Women's fantasies in the first trimester reflected both their emotional variability and their adjustment to a changed physical state. Fantasies of the baby tended to be global and less differentiated than later in pregnancy. They were primarily directed toward the task of incorporation, of letting the child or pregnancy into their lives.

> where am I with my quarter-of-an-incher? The ultimate in letting someone else in. I have an unfocused feeling, sometimes not feeling much at all about pregnancy, John, other relationships. Other times I feel incredibly vulnerable and bursting with love. See-saw. (Anna, 4 weeks)

While all the women had "felt ready" to conceive, the sense of themselves as mothers to a child of their own was not yet established. In the first trimester, women felt connected to their fetus in different ways. Anna felt an intuitive connection with her child even before conception. In the first trimester, she already had a strong feeling that her child was masculine (her child was indeed a boy), and she felt a powerful connection with him. She experienced this connection in the form of trust and willingness to "cooperate" with the pregnancy, whatever it entailed. Her freedom from incapacitating physical symptoms and her sense of intimate connection with her fetus combined to form an initial relatedness based on intuition, emotional receptivity, and merger. This allowed her to incorporate the pregnancy fairly easily. As pregnancy progressed, however, she had to work to develop a more individuated sense of herself to be able to mother her infant autonomously.

Katherine and Rachael, affirmed in their femininity by the event of pregnancy, felt "womanly" but not yet "motherly" in the first trimester. The connection to their child was felt in terms of allowing themselves to be more dependent and traditionally "female" while at the same time feeling concerned about the physical well-being of the fetus. Taking care of themselves was directly linked to taking care of the fetus. Katherine felt worried about having colds in the first months, Rachael found she had to give up jogging. Feelings of helplessness and being responsible blended together.

> I have fears of "Is my baby all right?"; fears of the baby being damaged. I feel so responsible, yet there is nothing I can do. (Katherine, 10 weeks)

For Linda, the first trimester proved most difficult. Preoccupied by managing her physical condition, she felt little maternal feeling in the first trimester at all.

> So far, I'm not feeling maternal, although I've looked forward to having a baby and generally love children. I definitely "know" I'm pregnant, but it's through the discomfort I feel I know this, not through the presence of maternal feeling. (Linda, 9 weeks)

For her, the incorporative aspects of early pregnancy in which mother and fetus are merged were traumatic. Extreme physical distress gave her the sense of being invaded by her fetus rather than joined with it. The question of which emotional or physical factors precipitated the severity of her physical condition is difficult to determine. Physical symptomatology occurs in interaction with psychological and social spheres.

Linda felt physically ill, felt guilty about being ill, and was frustrated with the impact of the illness on the rest of her life. The compounding factors led to problems in her sense of self-esteem and inhibited initial development of the prenatal maternal bond. Yet, once the fetal movements began, a shift in her physical condition and the clearer sense of her baby as separate from herself combined to promote a strong feeling of relatedness with her child. This feeling held throughout the rest of pregnancy, and she established a warm relationship with her infant after delivery.

The case of Linda is particularly interesting. The psychoanalytic literature addresses the pathological nature of hyperemesis in pregnancy, describing it as a symbolic, unconscious rejection of the child and the feminine role (Deutsch, 1944). Yet there is little material describing what it actually feels like for a woman to be experiencing this level of physical distress, nor is this condition evaluated in terms of its larger effects on a woman's life. Feeling ill, unable to work or go out, unable to eat or share meals with her husband, and held responsible for the severity of her condition, it is not surprising that Linda felt ambivalent about being pregnant and, initially, uncertain of her maternal feelings.

Thus, the first trimester brings with it a range of psychological effects. Heightened emotional sensitivity, mood changes, and a sense of separateness contribute to a subtle drawing away from usual concerns. It is as if the child within begins to make a definite, though still unstructured, space for itself in the life and thoughts of a woman long before its physical appearance either as a protruding belly or later as an actual newborn. The extraordinary subtlety of some of these shifts makes the nuances hard to catch. They flow gradually from one into the other until sudden nodal points are reached, such as the quickening, or the day the woman first puts on maternity clothes, or the first time an uninformed stranger asks if the woman is pregnant. The evolution of these changes is discussed in the next sections.

The Second Trimester

The main event of the second trimester, the appearance of fetal movements, or quickening, had great emotional significance for all the women in this study. Together with a lessening of physical symptoms and a corresponding increase in feelings of well-being, these months tended to be among the most satisfying of the pregnancy. This is probably the period Freud (1931) had in mind when, regarding the emotional calmness of pregnant women, he concluded that pregnancy must be a period during which women live out the bliss of having their basic instinctual wishes gratified by full satisfaction of the drive organization of the female procreative function. More recent investigations have revealed that the apparent calm of this period is relative (Benedek, 1950). Even during these months, the emotional disequilibrium caused by the stresses of pregnancy and the inherent danger of parturition remain as a source of tension requiring ongoing physiological adjustment and psychological adaptation.

Women in this study experienced the second trimester both as a time of greater satisfaction and as a period of continuing pressure to integrate the psychobiological processes of pregnancy. They described a sudden increase in emotional lability, a slackening of sexual interest, and continued intensification of internal imagery as characteristic of this period. For each woman, the appearance of the fetal movements was greeted with excitement and a greatly enhanced sense of the baby's aliveness and separateness. After brief adjustment to the novel sensations, women came to appreciate and derive reassurance from the fetal movements. In each case, the fetal movements were experienced as a means of communication with the baby. Sometimes the movements stimulated fantasies about the child or caused parents to attempt "conversations" with the fetus.

I want the movements so I can feel more in communication with the baby. I've had fantasies that the baby is a boy because there is so much movement. I've done a lot of daydreaming about boys and we did this superstitious way of testing the sex of the baby where you dangle a needle on a thread over your baby . . . It came out reading that it was a boy . . . (Rachael, 21 weeks)

My husband and I have a name for the fetus. When we talk about him, we call him "Felix." (Katherine, 16 weeks)

In this way, the quickening became a concrete step forward in the growing specificity of the pregnancy experience for each woman. Now, in addition to simply imagining the child, the fetal movements became a way of both imagining and feeling the child. It is striking that each woman interpreted this pivotal point of her pregnancy in terms of issues of special significance to her life. Anna, whose major preoccupation throughout pregnancy had to do with developing a sense of autonomy, felt alone and lonely in the first trimester. For her, the quickening gave her a sense of being supported in her pregnancy by the presence of this other being who was a part of this experience in a way no one else could be. When her baby began to move, she shifted from feeling "lonely" and the fear of being "taken over" by the pregnancy at 16 weeks to feeling like she and her baby were partners at 19 weeks.

I've been feeling lonely, but what has made it better this time is that I've felt support from "the other" in my body and know that we're in this together. An undercurrent from the beginning has been how alone one is in the pregnant state. I wanted someone in there with me to have hand in hand through it all. I feel now that someone [the baby] is. (Anna, 19 weeks)

Rachael's and Katherine's feelings were also reflective of their personal concerns. Rachael, the most professionally developed of the women in the study, experienced herself as doing a "good job" with her pregnancy when the fetal movements appeared. Katherine responded out of her newly affirmed sense of her body. She experienced the quickening in terms of, "This baby is developing properly, and I am developing properly along with it, as a woman should." For Linda, the quickening occurred approximately at the same time that amniocentesis revealed the sex of her child. Finding that she was to have the girl she had sex-determined for, and feeling the movements, produced a dramatic reversal in her feelings about the pregnancy. Instead of feeling invaded and taken over by a hostile force, she now interpreted her previous distress as the result of her prospective daughter's "feistiness."

Once the baby moved, I felt more personally attached. All of a sudden it was this moving baby in there instead of a shrimp. Then, when they called to tell me the results of the amniocentesis, and they said it was a girl first, I was overjoyed. I never doubted

> she would be healthy. I knew somebody was surviving. I knew she was just feisty.
> Since then, the pregnancy has taken on new meaning. I'm housing a baby, a child with
> a personality, instead of a monster and a fish. (Linda, 18 weeks)

When she reformulated some of her previous difficulties in terms of her daughter's vitality and activity, she found herself able to connect with her unborn child in a more differentiated way. While still physically uncomfortable, and occasionally resentful of her distress, she was now able to balance these feelings with the vivid sense of having a child of her own.

In this way, the more clearly felt presence of another inside themselves led to the development of an internal duality with consequences for the developing maternal bond. This finding is in keeping with previous theoretical writings (Chertok, 1973; Deutsch, 1944) which comment on the development of internal duality in pregnancy. They trace this duality throughout the experience of conception, pregnancy, and childbirth. Conception initially blends two separate entities into the unity of the fertilized ovum. This evolves into the psychosomatic unity/symbiosis of mother and fetus in the early stages of pregnancy. As pregnancy progresses, a more developed sense of internal duality is experienced and brought into focus by the fetal movements. From then on, mother and fetus become two foci in a dynamic field. Within this field, an expectant mother can accentuate either the sense of herself as united, as one with the fetus, or the sense of herself as separate from the fetus. These two positions have been interpreted in the literature as a progressive/active urge forward into the anticipated caretaking role and a progressive/passive move backward into sympathetic identification with the helpless infant. Both processes are seen as important for adequate development of the maternal role. Both active nurturing or caretaking behavior and empathic understanding of one's infant are viewed as the natural outcome of integrating these processes.

Women in this study found that conception and early pregnancy tended to affirm their "womanliness," but the appearance of the fetal movements furthered awareness of their "motherliness." Especially after quickening, feelings about their situation took on a dual perspective. Awareness of themselves became mixed in with speculation about the baby as a separate locus of needs and feelings.

> I wonder if the womb is really a quiet place. I wonder if I'm providing a comfortable
> place for the baby. I'm trying to understand why the kicking goes on . . . in my
> thoughts during the day, I talk to the baby and stroke my belly. I find myself relating
> to the baby as "little me." I wonder how I was as a little girl. I talk to it as "little
> Katherine." (Katherine, 19 weeks)

It is important to remember in this respect that the primary relation initiated with the fetus is composed of a relation with an imagined infant, i.e., a part of the self objectified in fantasy. It is only after delivery that the mother's fantasies about her child must give way to the growing reality of her child's personality.

Part of the satisfaction during this period may be linked to increasing familiarity with the pregnant state. As the abdomen enlarged and women started to wear maternity clothes sometime in the second trimester, the visibility of their condition contributed to feeling more "legitimate." As Katherine put it, "I'm feeling more and more comfortable being an expectant mother."

Yet changes in mood which began in the first trimester persisted and intensified in the second trimester. Every woman experienced herself as emotionally labile, subject to sudden changes in her intensity or pattern of emotional response. These changes occurred regardless of a woman's "prepregnancy" personality. Emotional lability increased as the second trimester progressed and remained evident throughout the rest of pregnancy.

> For days in the last 5 weeks I have been taken over by my emotions. Whatever the feelings—anger, death, etc.—I have been engulfed by the feeling. It just had its way with me until it was over. (Anna, 24 weeks)

> These last weeks I've felt more emotional than usual. After the third month, I felt my emotions were more normal, but now my emotions have resurfaced. (Rachael, 21 weeks)

Women in the present study were aware that their emotional response to given situations was at times exaggerated, but the knowledge did little to change the expression of feeling.

> At the same time there were gushes of emotion having to do with death. We went to buy a Christmas tree . . . I couldn't stand all those dead trees; I was just weeping in the Christmas tree lot over all those trees that had been cut down. And I was laughing at the same time, because I knew I was absolutely ridiculous. (Anna, 24 weeks)

The emotional lability was linked to a changing sense of self. The feeling of personal transformation, of new aspects of the self rising to the surface, was quite pronounced in the second and third trimesters. New emotional sensitivities carried over into dream life and fantasies stimulating an awareness of internal imagery which, for one woman, felt like an actual change in consciousness.

> I've felt there are levels of consciousness that I've been exposed to in my waking life and in dreams that are totally nonverbal. There have been some dreams that I've felt were astonishing, and they were at levels of perception that I've never known before.

But there has been no way to communicate them. There is no verbal or even cognitive translation. They are just other states. (Anna, 12 weeks)

Rachael, who was inclined to view initial changes in her dream life as reflective of hormonal changes, found the contents of her dreams thought-provoking. Her interpretation of them as compensatory for the aspects of her life that were changed by the pregnancy points to the pervasive psychological impact of the physical experience of pregnancy.

One thing that has been happening—and I attribute it just to hormonal changes—is that I have been having a lot of overt sexual dreams that have been surprising to me. I've never been a person who had a lot of graphic sexual dreams . . . and I've thought in addition to it just being kind of a hormonal thing that these dreams are kind of wish fulfilling. At times they even seem to avoid the reality of pregnancy. I've been dreaming of myself as effortlessly out jogging when I've had to give up jogging so I could feel more comfortable about being pregnant. In my dreams I jog hundreds of miles without feeling bad. And having all these sexual escapades, mostly with men from my past, which again feels like a piece of me that I am giving up and committing myself away from in a whole, deeper way through the pregnancy and marriage. (Rachael, 20 weeks)

Along with greater awareness of inner life, all the women experienced a continuation of earlier tendencies to be less interested in external events. It proved more difficult to concentrate or genuinely care about previous interests.

I've had a hard time working. I feel like sitting on the couch and waiting, staring at the wall. Waiting is like nothing interests me, nothing captures my attention. (Katherine, 17 weeks)

The preoccupying nature of pregnancy became more intense from a subjective point of view. Even though the women had adapted to the initial changes in awareness that were a part of the first trimester and strived to continue with their daily routine as usual, they found that their thoughts inevitably returned to their pregnancy.

I can never forget that I'm pregnant. It's something that totally preoccupies you. So there is this sense of distance from other people. Because you're experiencing something that is constant and pretty big and involves how you think about yourself as a person and your future and everything is up for grabs at that point. Everything leads you to look at it in a different way; I mean you look at everything in a different way. Or with the sense that it might change. (Linda, 22 weeks)

The sense of being more separate from others as a result of being pregnant, which women experienced in the first trimester, took on different dimensions in the second trimester after the fetal movements began.

Then there was the simultaneous feeling of isolation from others who did not share similar preoccupations and yet a sense of never being able to really be alone again because of the continuous presence of the fetus.

> Once the baby starts to move, you're never alone after that. You can't go away by yourself and be yourself, because you are—Somebody else is a part of you and somebody else is with you; and I know that it's a really big question at this point—in terms of the baby's conscious—But you aren't ever alone in the pregnancy after that, ever again; you're just not alone. (Linda, 24 weeks)

Fluctuations in sexual desire during this period, as well as the increased awareness of the fetus, led to concerns with the problem of integrating sexuality and motherhood. A number of factors affected how these concerns were viewed. Aside from physiological changes, the husband's response to his wife's attractiveness, historical antecedents in the mother's own psychosexual history, and concern over the safety of intercourse during pregnancy all contributed to the situation. Previously sexuality had been seen in terms of being "lovers" with one's husband. Now, the added dimension of self as mother and the presence of the fetus demanded integration.

All the women found themselves less sexually interested during the second trimester when these concerns first became more prominent. Katherine found herself thinking of sex as a more serious thing than before. Part of her felt some nostalgia for the time when sex had seemed more lighthearted and "fun." She worried about becoming "too maternal," yet found that she really was not as interested in making love as before. Rachael first experienced some conflict over these different aspects of her sexuality when she found herself missing the days when her husband affectionately called her "fox." Instead, he had taken to calling her "mom" or "mother"—even when she did feel sexually inclined. Somehow she found it difficult to feel "sexual" and "motherly" at the same time. Resolution of these concerns did not fully occur in pregnancy but continued after childbirth as part of the ongoing adjustment to parenthood.

Thus, the second trimester brought with it continuing psychological changes. Some of these involved an intensification of subtle changes already felt in the first trimester. Others represented more sudden shifts in response to new events like the quickening or the increased size of the abdomen.

The Third Trimester

The end of the second trimester and the beginning of the third blended together emotionally. It was somewhere in this period that all the women suddenly began to feel impatient with the pregnancy and the first thoughts about wanting it to end arose. Then, as the pregnancy neared conclusion, all the women began to find their interest shifting from internal preoccupation with themselves or the baby to active preparations for the birth. Called the "nesting instinct" in many books about pregnancy and motherhood, this was also clearly evident in the women of this study. As their interest shifted to these preparations, they suddenly found themselves feeling more detached from the fetus and focused on the labor and delivery itself. Throughout this trimester, dreams and fantasies continued to reflect the immediate concerns of impending motherhood and delivery. Emotional lability also continued as a regular feature of the pregnancy experience.

Toward the end of the second trimester and the beginning of the third, three of the women in this study found themselves preoccupied by not wanting to be alone. Each of them tried to stay as close to her husband as possible. Sometimes this translated into a constant need to know where he was and when he would return. Increased feelings of vulnerability and dependency that were a part of this need continued throughout the third trimester.

> I've been feeling so dependent on Tim, emotional dependency, physical dependency . . . I just have to know down to the last minute when he's going to be home: "You're 15 minutes late; why are you 15 minutes late?" Because all of a sudden you're aware that—it's almost like there you are in the nest, nurturing this baby and there's somebody else—Well, that isn't true for every woman, but in my case it—Having been that I was in school, I am not making money, so Tim is the person who is supporting us and he is out there in the world. . . . And I am sitting on the eggs back in the nest. So I've really needed to know when he is coming home, where he is. I've needed him by me. (Linda, 28 weeks)

> I get restless being in the house. Something about being home alone that is really distasteful to me. When I'm at home, I keep checking my watch to see when Bill will be home. I need him in the house in order to feel safe or to be able to work. It troubles me that I have this restlessness, that I can't stay put alone and at home. (Katherine, 27 weeks)

Feelings of impatience with the pregnancy began as early as the end of the second trimester for one woman. Two others experienced these feelings somewhat later in the third trimester. Linda, who had experienced such feelings very early in the pregnancy due to her physical difficulties, now found herself enjoying her pregnancy more than she had previously been able to do. For her, the desire to meet her baby after delivery rather than increased physical discomfort focused her attention on the end of pregnancy.

For the women who experienced an increase in physical symptoms in the third trimester, the pregnancy became a source of disaffection and irritability.

> I just feel awful. I'm physically uncomfortable; it's hard to walk and that's upsetting. I am constantly angry and upset about it. I thought pregnancy would not be uncomfortable, but I'm finding it is and no one understands. (Katherine, 29 weeks)

As their bodies became larger and larger, there appeared to be a loosening of body boundaries. Women had the sense of hardly recognizing themselves and feeling "lost" inside their pregnant bodies:

> feel like I've gotten so big. I don't want to be out there. I feel like I'm in everybody's way, like my stomach is between me and normal life. (Katherine, 29 weeks)

The changes happening to their bodies were reflected in a gradual reorientation to the physical aspects of pregnancy. Apprehension in early pregnancy was more focused on how the pregnancy would change them, their self-image, and their bodies. Then as pregnancy progressed, this more narcissistic preoccupation with the self began to incorporate preoccupation with the contents of their bodies, i.e., the baby. Women became concerned about what it felt like to be inside the womb. Now, in the third trimester, there was more tension in the balance between concern for the baby and anxiety about the self. Women began to feel more frustrated with having to subordinate their own well-being to that of the baby.

> At this point in pregnancy I feel like the baby is really becoming intrusive and there is really no escape. There is no measuring out my giving and my not giving. I have to be giving all the time. I mean I've had some illnesses and haven't been able to take medication, and I am awakened at night all the time instead of being able to sleep. I just don't feel like I have the space to get the strength I need to give. I'm tired of it and feel intruded upon by it. (Rachael, 29 weeks)

The desire to have the pregnancy over with increased under this pressure. It was further stimulated by growing curiosity about what the baby would actually be like once it was born. In the latter part of the second and the first part of the third trimester, the deepening affective tie with the fetus was reflected in shifting images in dreams and fantasies. Less differentiated images of the fetus evolved into images of a more fully formed baby. Women had begun to personify the fetus in the second trimester and this continued in the third. By this time, women were quite familiar with the fetal movements, had learned to differentiate various types of movement, and had imbued the movements with human characteristics. Linda, for example, thought she would have a strong, feisty child because there was so much movement, while Rachael thought she must be having a boy for the same reasons.

By the third trimester, these various interactions with the fetus led women to express a clear sense of having established a relationship with it. The fetal movements were seen as the basis of communication and interaction, a form of "conversation" between mother and child.

> There are times—I mean, feeling her kick is just miraculous to me. Especially lately. I sit in bed at night and watch this like thunder storm play across my belly. It's just amazing. Then there are times when I feel this like butterfly brush underneath my navel, and it's so clear to me that it's her hand, her fingers fluttering, one at a time across—underneath and across my belly. Which is just amazing to me; I just cannot comprehend that. And then she gets hiccups several times a day; that seems wondrous. I've also read somewhere that babies are fed within half an hour after the mother eats, and it's clear to me that her behavior will change. She'll start moving around and bumping and kicking, and then when I eat, she'll calm down. So I've started to feel a connection with her. I feel this real curiosity about what she is like. I keep thinking about wishing I had a camera in there to watch her, because she has such personality; I mean she has become such a being to me. (Linda, 32 weeks)

As the third trimester continued, however, dream images shifted again. This time threatening images of assault and rape, voyages of various types, and dreams picturing anxiety-provoking mother-child relations were common. Dreams of assault and rape were generally linked to fears of being assaulted, attacked, or torn open by the impending trauma of childbirth.

> I have been having bad dreams. They are graphic and horrible, like the Sharon Tate murders. The body is all cut up and the baby exposed. I also dream about battle scenes, soldiers, and war. (Anna, 35 weeks)

Dreams about going places by means of vehicles or natural forces as a phenomenon of the third trimester have been noted by other researchers (Colman & Colman, 1971; Kestenberg, 1978). These dreams are also associated with the anticipation of having the baby come out. Often the vehicle is a way of having the baby come out or is seen as a symbol of change from one state (expectant motherhood) to another (motherhood).

> I've had dreams about trying to go on a trip and that I had to pack the car and that I kept packing the car full of pillows; and I could never get them all in, they kept popping out, because I had all these pillows to stuff in. (Linda, 29 weeks)

Dreams involving scenes of mother-child relations were generally colored by anxiety.

Dreamt I was still pregnant—this wasn't my baby this was happening with. Anyway, somebody gave me a premature doll-like baby to take care of. I didn't feel responsible for it. I put it down, mislaid it. I went to a party and when I came home I couldn't find it. I panicked and finally found the baby among all these pillows. I didn't know what food it needed. I wondered, could I keep it alive on colostrum* until my own baby comes? (Rachael, 33 weeks)

In the last weeks of pregnancy, sleep became more and more fragmented due to increasing physical discomfort or restlessness. As a result, the boundary between sleeping and waking, between dreaming and reality, became blurred.

My sleep is very irregular now. I sleep 2 hours and then wake up. There is a lot of fuzziness between sleeping and waking. I'm unsure about what is a dream and what isn't. I have a sense of reality in my dreams. (Katherine, 36 weeks)

Then I had a dream that I had to escape from a house and I was absolutely terrified. I found this little, tiny rectangle through which I stuffed myself. I mean it was so tiny and I was just pushing myself out of this hole and it was very scary. It felt a lot like a birth and delivery to me, or a labor dream. It began to get a little confusing about whether I was dreaming about my feelings about what was happening or whether the dreams were what the baby was feeling. (Linda, 30 weeks)

This sense of confusion eventually began to extend to previous feelings of connectedness with the fetus. Suddenly women in this study felt less attached to the baby and more preoccupied with the imminence of childbirth. Feelings of detachment from the baby at times even took on a rejecting quality.

I am not feeling connected to the baby. I don't feel in tune with it now. I feel rejecting of him. I can't get past that, there is only delivery now. (Anna, 35 weeks)

Fluctuations in energy experienced physically as alternations between fatigue and bursts of energy were mirrored psychologically. Feelings of lassitude vied with restlessness.

*Colostrum is the pre-milk fluid secreted in the breasts during pregnancy. After the birth, this is the first food the baby gets from the mother. It contains antibodies which are a part of his defense system against infection. The true milk does not come into the breasts until the third day. (Taken from *Dictionary of Pregnancy, Childbirth and Contraception*, Mayflower Books, 1971)

> Sometimes I feel passive and calm, like a quietness that comes over me. Then I feel like I don't know what to do with my energy. (Rachael, 34 weeks)

Frequently, bursts of energy were translated into activity as women started making more active preparations for their babies, such as purchasing baby clothes or buying baby furniture. Housecleaning and ordering also bore witness to this nesting instinct. To some extent, this activity served defensive purposes as women preferred to keep their thoughts occupied with preparations for the baby rather than with fears about delivery.

> Someone asked me recently if I was looking forward to the day. I find I don't think about the event. My energy goes into preparations. (Katherine, 32 weeks)

At the same time, nesting activities consolidated awareness of the baby as a separate, concrete entity. This accords with Helene Deutsch's (1945) view that "nesting" serves an adaptive function by helping women prepare in concrete ways for the impending separation from the fetus.

As the third trimester drew to a close, women had fleeting thoughts that they had taken on a lifetime responsibility of having a child. A renewed sense that the end of pregnancy meant a significant life change emerged quite clearly.

> I have feelings of both wanting and not wanting this child, of not wanting my life changed, or not wanting all these obligations. (Katherine, 33 weeks)

Thus, the physical discomfort of the third trimester spawned psychological parallels. Increased irritability, impatience, and new feelings of detachment from the fetus coupled with eagerness to see their child after its birth emotionally prepared the women to let go of their child in childbirth.

Labor and Delivery

The experience of labor and delivery was perceived as an overwhelming event by all the women in this study. Quite apart from the physical difficulties which they encountered to varying degrees, the drama and emotional impact of childbirth was an event without parallel in their previous experience.

All of the women had physically and emotionally prepared themselves for childbirth with the help of various psychoprophylactic or natural childbirth methods (e.g., Lamaze, Read, and Bradley). These methods stress that pain is a perception as well as a physical response. As such, pain is considered to be emotionally reactive and subject to psychological control. Factors such as fear and anxiety are seen as causing tension, thereby increasing pain during childbirth. Psychoprophylaxis seeks to regulate these factors by providing information and teaching the use of special relaxation techniques aimed at producing psychological analgesia during labor and delivery.

In the past decade, the popularity of these methods, first developed in Europe, has dramatically increased in the United States. Indeed, there has been a tendency in some areas of the country to view natural childbirth as the only acceptable way to deliver a child. Consequently, the inability to deliver a child in this way has become open to being interpreted as a personal failure to perform adequately in this most quintessentially female act. In fact, the Pavenstadt (1959) study of the relationship between maturity and childbirth concludes that the ease and smoothness of childbirth is unrelated to the maturity of the parturient woman's personality. Some of the most immature mothers have the easiest confinements, demonstrating that personality factors other than maturity are involved in childbirth. Exactly what these are is still unknown. Nonetheless, the women in this study were representative of the movement favoring natural childbirth and tended to view labor and delivery as a time when they would be able to test themselves personally.

The ability to tolerate childbirth with little or no medical intervention was linked to self-esteem in various ways. Linda, who was informed ahead of time that she would need a Caesarean section, described her distress very aptly.

> I mean I just feel like here is the perfect ending to this perfectly lousy pregnancy! I did it wrong from the beginning; I'm doing it wrong now. You know, there is this real prevailing thing in the Bay Area that there is a right way to do everything. You nurse your baby; you deliver in the ABC [Alternative Birth Center]. You never take any pills during pregnancy; you never have medication during delivery. So the fact that I will be having a C-section just blows me away. (Linda, labor and delivery)

She had hoped to use the experience of labor and delivery to learn something about herself and perhaps recoup some of the losses in self-esteem which had been a part of her pregnancy experience.

> All of these things that I had prepared myself to deal with and I thought, I'm really gonna overcome—I'm gonna triumph over pain and I'm gonna decide I'm a brave person, that I really could go through this [labor and delivery], and won't that be wonderful? It will affect the rest of my life and I'll like myself. Of course, I was scared, too. But I was looking forward to the chance. I was looking forward to the struggle, because I wanted—really wanted to learn something about myself from that. (Linda, labor and delivery)

After her initial disappointment was worked through, she was in fact able to feel excited about the delivery and even about the first stages of labor. When her water broke, she described it as "Christmas and Halloween together, and New Year's." Once in the hospital, she faced a number of unwelcome standard obstetrical procedures with patience and humor and greeted her newborn with intense excitement. Rachael, who also delivered by Caesarean section, had similar feelings of loss about not being able to fulfill her hopes for a natural childbirth. She did, however, experience labor and felt satisfied with her performance during this time. She did describe her feelings of loneliness during labor.

> My husband was with me throughout labor and delivery, so it wasn't that I was physically alone . . . yet the intensity of the experience that I was having was real isolating and it was hard to believe that anybody else was really there for what was going on with me. When I would be awake and unable to sleep for contractions and my husband would be asleep, I would feel very angry and alone and abandoned. (Rachael, labor and delivery)

As labor wore on with little relief, Rachael found herself losing touch with normal reality.

> I felt like I was at times during that whole 2 days kind of out of my body and out of contact, in another world. (Rachael, labor and delivery)

As soon as her baby was born, however, she was overcome with relief and euphoria. She described herself as "flying" and in love with her baby, her husband, and the people who were caring for her in the hospital.

Anna and Katherine also had long labors. Anna needed some medical intervention during her labor and delivery, but she was able to remain in control with the help of her husband and a friend who acted as her coaches. For her, labor involved a reorientation of priorities. Prior to labor, she had felt some resentment about the secondary role assigned to the mother during parturition. Now, in labor, she realized that she was a vehicle for her child's birth and she was able to fully accept her own role as a vital but nonetheless supporting one.

> There was a real strong moment early in labor where I realized this was not my show. I had a supporting role here; a vital one, for sure, but this was his show, it wasn't about me. I wasn't the star here. I had always thought these people so self-effacing and self-sacrificing; that's how I saw that kind of talk before. But obviously, when you're coming from that point of view, well . . . it's a completely different perspective. 'Cause you're the mother. You are the mother, you are the vehicle for this child. (Anna, labor and delivery)

Anna used her insight to help her in labor, concentrating on cooperating with each contraction, viewing each contraction as a step along the way to delivering her child. She found that her concern for her baby focused itself on maintaining a sense of connection with it.

> I remember often sort of keeping this channel open. I mean it wasn't anything I did; it was just a feeling I had about keeping this channel open to the baby. And that going through this birth, he would do just fine if I could just keep in touch with him. It was totally nonverbal. (Anna, labor and delivery)

Her sense of connection with her baby was such that she didn't even ask whether it was a boy or a girl. She knew her child would be a boy. Yet she had not anticipated further what he would look like. She found herself surprised by the physical beauty of her child.

> I didn't even ask what it was. I knew he was a boy. But when I opened my eyes, he was there and he was very calm and looking around, wide-eyed, and I was just suddenly astonished by how gorgeous he was. I hadn't pictured what he would look like. I just hadn't thought about it throughout the whole pregnancy. (Anna, labor and delivery)

This oversight on Anna's part is actually more or less characteristic of the other mothers as well. Their tie to the fetus is primarily affective and is less concerned with the physical attributes of the child. This allows for the widest receptivity to any number of possibilities. While two of the mothers in this study admitted that they needed some time after delivery to know and develop feelings of love for their child, all of the mothers described a "visceral" or gut connection with their child which was independent of the more developed feelings referred to as "love."

Although Katherine was able to have the natural childbirth she had planned on, she found herself critical of her performance. Interestingly enough, her description of her experience was quite different from how she appeared throughout labor to others. Both the midwife and her friends congratulated her on her endurance and stoicism, yet her subjective experience of labor and delivery revealed a more fragile sense of herself.

> I realized I felt ashamed, not proud of myself with respect to labor and delivery. The midwife said I should feel proud, but I knew the pain was more than I could bear. I looked like I was holding on, but inside I knew that somewhere along the line I crumbled. I was suffering. I had my limits. (Katherine, labor and delivery)

It is interesting that even Katherine, who had achieved the coveted experience of "natural" medication-free childbirth, was ultimately not satisfied with her performance. This would certainly suggest that something about the act of giving birth may indeed be becoming linked to impossibly high standards which women find difficult to fulfill. One of Katherine's friends talked about this, suggesting that childbirth was the female equivalent of male "machismo," requiring a stoicism and tolerance for pain which went beyond average limits.

Thus, labor and delivery proved a time of critical transition and challenge, taking women to the limits of their endurance and involving them in a process all of them saw as awesome. It is also clear that the value of preparation before labor and delivery does indeed lie in its power to provide women with knowledge and techniques that help them control the discomfort of labor and maintain some mastery of the situation.

Postpartum

The continued intensity of feeling shortly after childbirth came as a surprise to the women in this study. Three of them in particular found themselves having extreme moods of elation or depression, depending on interactions with their new baby. This seemed especially true of feelings connected to the nursing relationship.

> And I went through—it was really like a roller coaster ride. I was either at the top, ecstatic, or I was just plummeting to the bottom, in despair. I just didn't know any intermediate feelings sometimes. When a feeding would go well, I would feel just blissful. And when it didn't—either the milk didn't let down or he didn't suck well or something went wrong—I was just in despair. (Anna, postpartum)

Rachael also described herself as having unstable moods right after delivery. She found herself crying a lot and also feeling a lot of live and strong symbiotic feelings with the baby and with her husband. The intensity of these emotions amazed her. She remembered how, before delivery, she had been determined to not let her new identity as a mother consume her. Now, after delivery, she wanted nothing else than to be with her child.

> I didn't realize how vulnerable and dependent I would feel after delivery. I was just overflowing with feelings. That was a shock, how changed and moved I felt during this period. I remember a couple of weeks before delivery I was saying, "I really don't want to let the baby affect my life that much; I really don't want to give up my complete identity to the baby; I think I'm gonna be able to go out and do things when the baby's a couple of weeks old and leave it with someone else." And that was just really off-base from how I felt for a long time after the birth. I just felt very transformed. I felt like I just wanted to be in my house with my husband and my child and just sit and look at each other all the time. (Rachael, postpartum)

While intense preoccupation with the new baby was typical of all the women, two of them felt less immediately certain that they loved their child. They found that their feelings developed more slowly as they got to know their child better.

> I worried that I didn't feel like I loved her when she was born. I couldn't connect with anything that felt like love. I had loved her so much when she was within me, now she was outside and I didn't know how I felt about her. Surprised I wasn't gushing. Then, a little later, I realized I really loved her, 3 or 4 weeks later, when her personality was more definite, more responsive. (Katherine, postpartum)

For these women, feelings of attachment, of love, came as a response to a more distinct sense of their child's personality.

Summary

From these findings, it is evident that the psychological experience of pregnancy is a complex mix of many variables. Wide variation in individual response to the physical aspects of pregnancy is further reflected in different types of emotional adaptation. Yet certain central unifying themes can be demonstrated. It seems clear that much of the emotional constellation during pregnancy is related to the unique relationship developed with the fetus. The emotional bond with the fetus develops with surprising rapidity after conception. This bond deepens and becomes more differentiated as pregnancy develops so that women have feelings of identity with the fetus as delivery approaches. These in turn stimulate readiness and eagerness to take on the maternal role in partnership with the actual baby. The emotional lability that appears as a feature of psychological life throughout pregnancy seems geared to extending a woman's receptivity to the wide fluctuations in mood and unstable sense of self that are a part of early infancy.

In addition to emotional changes during pregnancy, the birth of a child heralds changes in the matrix of social relations that surround the expectant mother. Reorientations of these relations and an examination of their importance for the mother are the subject of the next chapter.

6

Pregnancy: Its Psychosocial Effects

Overview

Environmental or psychosocial influences as well as individual psychology affect the overall constellation of the pregnancy experience. Just as the child is born into a finely interwoven network of preexisting relationships, so the expectant mother lives imbedded in her world of relationships. This is so prior to becoming pregnant, during the course of pregnancy, and after the child is born. As pregnancy progresses and women become increasingly dependent on their environment, they become increasingly susceptible to its influence. The environment gains in significance, especially at the level of interpersonal interaction, precisely because pregnancy is accompanied by heightened sensitivities and new vulnerabilities. Physical or emotional changes often require some external validation or recognition to become set into the pattern which the expectant mother comes to identify as uniquely her own.

Women in this study found themselves simultaneously more withdrawn from their environment and more dependent on it. The newness and the importance of being pregnant left women unsure at times about how to evaluate their experience in terms of what was unique to them and what was a predictable part of pregnancy. Consequently, they developed a sense of themselves in conversation with others as well as through internal reflection. This chapter presents these women's experience of pregnancy as it affected their environment and also takes up the way the environment affected them.

Conception

As mentioned in the previous chapter, the decision to conceive a child was largely determined by the perceived stability of the marital tie. Each woman in this study found that, as the idea to have a child gathered momentum, she began to look differently at her relationship with her husband. Generally, two processes were identified as important. Foremost was that of attachment, or the security and commitment of the marital bond. Second was that of mutuality, or the possibility for nurturing roles to be reversed as needed so that the husband could be perceived as being capable of caring for and nurturing the wife as she cared for and nurtured the fetus within her.

Prior to conception, all four women found issues of dependency and trust mixed in with their thoughts about having a baby. Three of them expressed this as a more or less conscious willingness to contemplate, at least temporarily, a more dependent position in relation to their husbands than had previously been the case. Katherine expressed this most clearly:

> There was a real shift in my feelings which started when I was trying to get pregnant. Basically, I felt more and more willing to be dependent. (Katherine, conception)

One woman, on the other hand, experienced issues of trust and dependency from a different perspective at this stage. Like the other women, she had evaluated her decision to conceive in the context of her perception of her marital relationship. Unlike them, she felt she also needed a clearer, more separate sense of herself. Before becoming pregnant, and definitely throughout the pregnancy itself, she emphasized her growth away from dependency on others and toward greater autonomy for herself.

> It [having a baby] was an impetus to me. I felt that it had to do with growing up. And growing up in my relationship with my husband. Separating and individuating, that's what growing up seemed to me to be about. It had to do with being on my own and doing this myself. (Anna, conception)

Conception itself was seen as a confirmation of the relationship between husband and wife. The event was viewed with pleasure and satisfaction, regardless of whether or not conception was accompanied by profound feeling at the time. Anna experienced conception as an ecstatic moment of union with her husband, while Katherine recalled being tired the night conception probably occurred; yet both women felt confirmed in their commitment to the marriage.

> So I had in my mind the month I wanted to get pregnant; it just seemed like the right time. And I didn't use birth control this time and I knew when I got pregnant. And it was a full moon. And it was just an ecstatic, joyful—I felt like I was bringing in. And that was it. (Anna, conception)

> So we knew it was a really right time in our life to do it [have a baby], career-wise and emotionally and in terms of the stability we felt we had. It was a nice time, sort of a romantic thing to be making love to have a baby, though probably the actual night of

conception was not anything special, other than that we knew we wanted to make a child. But we both felt really good, knowing that we had a baby coming. (Rachael, conception)

Except for Anna, who was not working when she became pregnant, the other women in this study timed conception in careful coordination with such external factors as career goals and study plans.

I was trying to finish a master's degree at the time and we had it all planned down to the last month, in terms of trying to get pregnant. We didn't try to get pregnant until it would leave enough time for me to finish my classes and my thesis. (Linda, conception)

These women were not only committed to their marriage and to becoming mothers but were also committed to their professional life. The requirements of this aspect of their lives became a significant variable in planning when to have a child and remained a source of anxiety and concern throughout pregnancy. As the realities of pregnancy and the realities of work began to impinge reciprocally on each other, each woman began to deal with the difficulties and complications of integrating these two separate sides of her life. The extent of physical symptomatology and emotional changes resulting from pregnancy, as well as the gradually widening social awareness of their pregnancy, were important factors in shaping the process of integrating work and motherhood.

For these women, conception represented not only personal readiness and interpersonal commitment, but also reflected ongoing concern for integrating personal and professional goals.

The First Trimester

After conception, feelings of closeness in the marriage continued in the early weeks of pregnancy, yet new anxieties about the husband as support and partner in the pregnancy emerged. Perhaps some of these feelings were linked to the growing realization that the husband could not totally participate in the pregnancy. Subtle feelings about being pregnant could not always be communicated, and the somatic symptoms of pregnancy obviously could not be shared. These feelings of being in some way alone in the pregnancy were more pronounced in three of the women. It is also true that the sense of being pregnant, of carrying another life within oneself, focused women's thoughts on their husbands with increased intensity. The husband's disposition toward them seemed of particular importance as women began to feel the early effects of pregnancy. Some women, like Katherine, began to question their husbands about the extent of support they could expect. In Katherine's case, the questions came out of an increased sense of vulnerability and dependency.

> I asked him questions like, Would he be there? Would he provide? Would he play with the child? He felt I was accusing him, but I still think it will be hard to do all I need to do. (Katherine, 8 weeks)

The realization that pregnancy was principally the woman's experience, whatever the previous sharing of stereotyped sex roles within the couple had been, took various forms. Two women experienced this distinction with some feelings of anger and resentment. Linda, suffering extreme physical discomfort, expressed this most keenly.

> I've gone through a period of resenting my husband for not being pregnant and not having to share in the nausea and discomfort. It's been hard to give up the notion of sharing equally in this child, at least as far as carrying and bearing and nursing it are concerned. (Linda, 7 weeks)

The other two women felt this in a more muted way. Shortly after conception, Anna wondered, for example, how she could communicate her certainty about being pregnant to her husband, who felt less sure than she was. She realized she could not give him that certainty quite simply because he couldn't feel what she felt.

> He didn't believe I was pregnant until I got a test. Even then, he didn't feel it was real. He didn't have any external manifestation of proof. And I knew inside; I had my proof, but it didn't work for him. Even after the test, the anxiety recurred for him. He just couldn't believe it, 'cause he didn't see it and he didn't feel it the way I felt it. (Anna, 5 weeks)

In this way, needs and concerns surfacing in the first trimester in connection with the couple's relationship were already indicative of future concerns later in pregnancy. Issues of attachment and mutuality present prior to and at the time of conception continued to be reflected in the first trimester.

Physical symptoms and feelings of separateness or aloneness began to carry over into social relations with surprising rapidity as women adjusted to the first trimester. Generalized fatigue, feelings of lassitude and subtle psychological reorientation, and the sense of being somehow different by virtue of being pregnant made social relations more difficult at first.

> to be with my friends, just to talk, to exchange the time of day takes so much effort because there is no way I can transmit—translate—what is going on inside. It isn't

verbal. It isn't even something I have an understanding of in my head. It is lonely; it is really lonely. (Anna, 5 weeks)

Gradually, as the women adjusted to the new feelings, they were able to resume social activity.

It's become easier for me to come back out and be with people; and it's become not such an effort. I guess I've become more comfortable with the fact that this [sense of withdrawal] is going on. (Anna, 10 weeks)

Except for Linda, who suffered unusual distress starting very early in pregnancy, the other women continued with their routines. As long as the pregnancy was not yet visible to others, couples had the choice of whom to tell. Close friends and family were the first to know. For the rest, the pregnancy still had an intimate, almost secret feel about it. At the same time, women began to feel that they had entered on an experience of universal proportions which united them to a collective past of female experience. All of the women in this study felt this at different times in the pregnancy. Anna mentioned it first, early in pregnancy; the other women tended to feel this more in the second or third trimesters. For Anna, it took the form of belonging to a new group, that of mothers and babies.

So many babies and pregnant women around! Nobody can tell, but I'm part of the tribe. (Anna, 9 weeks)

Linda, who was the most physically incapacitated of the women by the effects of pregnancy, was forced to curtail many of her previous activities and felt quite isolated at this stage. She found herself deeply resenting the images of pregnancy as a period of blissful contentment which she had internalized. Her personal experience was so dissonant from the cultural stereotype that she felt betrayed and angry. In her distress, she contacted both her mother and her sister to discuss what she called the "darker side" of pregnancy. To her surprise, she found that her sister had also experienced difficulties, although she had not mentioned them before.

My sister and mother both wrote to me with excitement about how wonderful it is to be pregnant. This didn't describe my experience at all, so I wrote to tell them how sick and tired and frustrated I've been. Both of them have written back in a way that lets me know they understand this darker side of pregnancy. My sister even shared some of the difficulties she had had when she was pregnant that she never told me about before. (Linda, 9 weeks)

Her sister's earlier lack of candor is in keeping with findings from other studies (Chertok, 1969; Colman & Colman, 1971; Leifer, 1980), which suggest that women are generally reluctant to reveal the full extent of their distress during pregnancy and consistently tend to rate their own experience as "average" almost regardless of their difficulties. In addition, Arthur and Libby Colman (1971) have written about the "amnesia" which seems to overtake the experience of pregnancy in the memory of many women after childbirth, making it difficult to recall actual feelings of distress or anxiety experienced at the time. While her sister's admission of her own difficulties with pregnancy comforted Linda, she still continued to feel upset when she heard others around her talk about the "bloom" and "bliss" of pregnancy.

The other women also contacted their mothers, but did not speak of being particularly close to them. At this stage of pregnancy, all the women felt themselves to be more dissimilar than similar to their mothers. There was a tendency to view their mothers as not especially warm or sympathetic either in terms of childhood memories or in terms of the present pregnancy. Women did wonder if the pregnancy would affect their relationship with their mothers, but they saw it more as something that would happen later in pregnancy or after childbirth rather than at this stage in the first trimester. It should be recalled that all the women in this study had mothers living outside the Bay Area, which may contribute to some of the feelings of distance that the women expressed.

The integration of work and maternity in the first trimester depended greatly on the extent to which physical symptoms interfered with the ability to carry on usual routines. Katherine and Rachael continued working as planned, although they felt tired most of the time and occasionally nauseated as well. Both of them did find themselves slowing down after work fairly early in the pregnancy. Linda, as already mentioned, was unable to continue with her studies. She spent most of her time at home and felt quite frustrated at this turn of events. It meant that she would not be able to finish her thesis or continue with classes. This only added to her ambivalence about being pregnant.

In a study of need achievement (Lindgren, 1976), it was found that expectant mothers had the lowest need achievement scores compared with samples of nonpregnant female students. These results were considered to be consistent with previous research and with expectations based on common sense and everyday impressions. In comparing nonstudent expectant mothers with nonpregnant female students, the study failed to consider the special relationship of achievement and time in the academic community. Certainly at the student level the two are linked together by class schedule and graduation deadlines. A totally different sense of time applies in most work situations. The lessening of need achievement in nonstudent expectant mothers would simply not entail the same consequences as would a similar change in expectant mothers who were also students.

For example, the intense frustration of finding herself incapacitated and unable to proceed with her academic plans was derived primarily from Linda's need for achievement within an academic framework. She had carefully timed the sequence of conception, pregnancy, and delivery to coincide with her academic schedule. The frustration of this plan by her unanticipated response to pregnancy wreaked considerable havoc with her self-esteem. In fact, her undiminished need for achievement in the professional sphere of her life made acceptance of her situation that much more difficult, especially early in the pregnancy.

Katherine, who struggled with similar concerns, although she was less physically taxed than Linda, began to feel this conflict later in pregnancy. There is little doubt that pregnancy tends to lessen a woman's interest in everyday external matters, but the extent to which her long-term goals recede from view is less clear. Both Katherine and Linda experienced the pregnancy as making frustrating inroads on their progress in developing themselves professionally. While these women did experience a temporary shift in need achievement during pregnancy, it appears that long-term need-achievement goals were not eclipsed by pregnancy.

In this way the first trimester already brought a number of changes to the expectant mother's interpersonal world. While the pregnancy confirmed the commitment of the marital relationship, new concerns about the husband as a partner in the pregnancy arose. Pregnancy also accentuated gender differences which had previously been less significant in the relationship. Fluctuations in desire for and interest in usual social activities led to changes in social relationships. Relationships with family, particularly with mothers, took on different significance. In general, the women in this study tended to see themselves as different from their mothers. Difficulties in the integration of work and maternity already made themselves felt in the first trimester. The extent of the difficulties at this stage was dependent on the expectant mother's adjustment to the physical effects of pregnancy.

The Second Trimester

The second trimester brought further changes to the marital relationship, to relationships with family and friends, and to the process of integrating personal and professional concerns. The interaction of physical and psychological effects continued to play a part in shifting interpersonal dynamics. A decrease in physical symptoms, the appearance of fetal movements, and growing external visibility of the pregnancy made the pregnancy easier to share with others. At the same time, feelings of internal preoccupation, increased feelings of vulnerability, and greater needs for affiliation sometimes left the women feeling critical of their relationship with their husband and closer to other women. The second trimester also prompted the women's interest in role rehearsal with other children in anticipation of caring for a child of their own. The visibility of the pregnancy toward the middle and end of the second trimester suddenly brought the pregnancy into the sphere of work relations in a new way contributing to further integration of work and motherhood.

For the women in this study, the marital relationship continued to be of central importance in the second trimester. Changes in physical appearance brought out greater needs for reassurance and stimulated anxiety about remaining sexually attractive to their husbands.

> My belly feels odd, like a grapefruit. I need more reassurance. My husband asked me about my nipples. Are they supposed to be that big? I worry about him being turned off. (Katherine, 16 weeks)

Women also experienced wanting more attention from their partners, as if their own preoccupation with their unborn child needed to be mirrored in some way by similar preoccupation on the part of their husbands. Katherine was able to say this clearly. For Linda, it came out in dream form:

> It feels like he [husband] is not as interested as I want him to be. I want him to be more attentive to me, to cater to me a little. (Katherine, 16 weeks)

> I dreamed about my mother and my husband. In the dream each of them were nurturing and taking care of me, although there was no interaction between the two of them. (Linda, 14 weeks)

Linda's dream placed her at the center of preoccupation of both her mother and her husband. In fact, Linda's unusual physical suffering, especially in the first four months of pregnancy, did require extra care and support. There had been plans for her to return home and be nursed by her mother, but she decided she did not feel well enough to travel. Instead, her mother came to California, arriving a few weeks after this dream.

The tendency to feel more introverted during the second trimester was not without impact on the marital relationship. While women longed for added attention and reassurance from their husbands, they also felt somewhat distant from them. This was especially true for three of the women and less the case for one. It is a striking finding of this study that three women found themselves feeling increasingly separate and even angry with their husbands during exactly the same time period. These feelings occurred from approximately 21 to 24 weeks into the pregnancy. They reached a peak at this time before gradually declining and being replaced by renewed feelings of closeness to the husband during the third trimester.

The precise source of these feelings is difficult to define. Perhaps women were themselves internally preoccupied, but from this new internal vantage point perceived their husbands as being less available. Perhaps husbands actually were less available. Increased emotional lability and dependence on the part of their wives may have stirred anxieties in them that they were best able to handle by being more withdrawn. Either way, the women felt suddenly more alone and isolated.

> I've been very angry with my husband. I've started to feel very alone in this pregnancy. I've had to carry the burden and the meaning of being pregnant all by myself. I've had such angry thoughts that I find myself making silent threats about leaving him. I feel so upset that he's just not as involved in this process as me. (Katherine, 20 weeks)

Another source for this phenomenon may be that, as women experienced their bodies in new and essentially female ways during pregnancy, they felt themselves to be more separate from their husbands, who might be sympathetic to their experience but could not fully comprehend it.

> I've continued to feel angry and resentful with Tim, that he isn't carrying the baby. I feel a growing separation from men. I feel interest from them, but still a lot of isolation. (Linda, 23 weeks)

The reality of being suddenly more vulnerable and in need of relying on their husband may also have triggered anger and anxiety.

> I've felt a lot of anger, incredible anger. Rage, with—mostly with John. There have been times when I just couldn't stand to be alone and I would want him to stay home. (Anna, 24 weeks)

Finally, since these feelings peaked shortly after the appearance of fetal movements, it should be considered that the more concrete reality of the baby experienced via the fetal movements may have suddenly brought the reality of motherhood into sharper focus. The newly felt existence of this child most emphatically demonstrated that henceforth their lives were no longer completely their own.

> I knew that pregnancy would bring a lot of changes, but recently I've felt a sense of loss and grieving which I attribute to the changes this will mean for me and for my husband [the arrival of a new person to take care of]. I feel anxious about being depended on by a baby and about my being more dependent on Tim as I become more tied to the home while caring for the baby. (Linda, 23 weeks)

A noteworthy exception to this finding was Rachael's experience. Unlike the other women in this study, Rachael did not experience increased feelings of anger with her husband during these particular weeks. She did briefly experience a period of tearfulness, during which she cried about the distance she felt suddenly opening up between them; but her feelings were short-lived, muted in comparison with the other women, and reflected no anger. This modulation of her feelings may have stemmed from the special relationship she enjoyed with her husband. He was unusually involved with her during pregnancy and tended to worry about being excluded from full participation in her experience. They were a remarkably close couple throughout pregnancy and remained so postpartum. Once the child was born, James even assumed half-time care of the infant.

Aside from this particularly stressful period, the middle trimester of pregnancy also had its special moments for husband and wife. This was generally the time when couples invented names for the fetus and attempted to carry on "conversations" with it. Anticipation of a baby led to discussions about the couple as a family and to hopeful plans for the future. Katherine moved to a new house; and other couples began thinking about which room would become the baby's.

Relationships with friends and family were important during this time, both as a source of support and in the way of trying out new roles. Women continued to reflect on their relationship with their mothers but did not express particular closeness with their mothers at this point. Of the women in this study, Rachael probably felt closest to her mother, but even she expressed this in the less personal terms of feeling a "generational connection" rather than a personally shared role identification. She saw her mother as having been the less nurturing one of her parents and hoped to be different herself. At the same time, her first thoughts that she might not be remembering her mother entirely accurately surfaced at this time. Thinking about this, she wondered how it would be to see her mother with her own child and thought it might give her some clues about the actual nature of her relationship with her mother during her own infancy.

> My first memory is of lying in a crib. I must have been about 2½. I was cold, but I didn't know how to say it. I cried and nobody came. My mother put her foot down and wouldn't let my father come in and walk me to sleep as he usually did. I wonder

about what kind of mother I had. She seems like an obsessive lady who put all her drive and intelligence into homemaking. It will be interesting to see her with my child and find out about how accurate I am. (Rachael, 23 weeks)

While Katherine had wanted more contact with her mother since the beginning of her pregnancy, she had been disappointed. Her initial call to her mother in the first month of her pregnancy had been an undefined call for reassurance. She had no specific concerns to discuss with her mother, and the conversation had remained vague and unsatisfying. Her second call proved no more gratifying. She had more specific questions to discuss this time, but found her mother unwilling to say more than that she was sure things would be different for Katherine than they had been for her. By the second trimester, Katherine decided not to contact her mother with her anxieties or to talk with her at all until they could see each other over Christmas. Instead, she thought about an older friend who had more of the "ideal" qualities she hoped to emulate. She described this friend as a "surrogate" mother who was "round, maternal, and always ready with a kiss or a hug." She remembered her own mother being this way with her when she had been younger, but then things had changed. The closeness was lost.

I remember her [my mother] being very loving and good to me as a little child; it's just that she understood me less and less as I grew up. (Katherine, 19 weeks)

Like Rachael, Katherine wondered how it would be to see her mother with her child. In her speculations, she drew a comparison between herself and her mother which actually aligned them with each other.

I'm curious to see how she will respond to her grandchild. Will she pick it up naturally or be nervous as she is with other children? I guess I'm nervous with kids, too, like her. I feel I may break them or something. (Katherine, 19 weeks)

Linda, who did not feel "particularly close" with her mother during pregnancy, nonetheless had a pleasant visit with her during this time. Her mother bought her her first maternity blouse and Linda experienced this gesture as "very sentimental and nice." Anna began to look forward to having her mother see her in her pregnant state.

Thus, the second trimester introduced new nuances into the women's relationships with their mothers. In the first trimester they had felt themselves to be mostly dissimilar from their mothers and tended to see their mothers as not especially good role models for themselves. Now, in the second trimester, women still expressed dissatisfaction with aspects of their relationships with their mothers, but they were more inclined to consider modifications in their previous views. The possibility that they might potentially be like their mothers in some ways when they themselves became mothers, or the desire to ascertain the accuracy of their ideas about their mothers, now generated curiosity about seeing their mothers in the grandmother role. Feelings of not being as "close" to their mothers as they would ideally have liked were significant at different emotional levels. While these feelings were certainly expressive of the actual nature of their relationships with their mothers, the desire for a more nurturing mother figure at this time may also be linked to expectant mothers' increased needs and wishes to be nurtured themselves.

All of the women talked about the importance of friendships, particularly with other women. Feelings of being special, of needing and enjoying extra attention, went hand in hand with feeling physically more at ease and more energetic in the second trimester.

> Now that the first trimester is over, I've felt pretty special with my friends. They've all been real nice to me and given me special attention, like I've sort of been in a place of honor. (Linda, 20 weeks)

As women began to look more pregnant, the first inquiries about their condition were met with pleasure.

> Other people are beginning to notice. People are becoming interested in a really nice way. I talk about it more eagerly, I feel more legitimate now in the second trimester. (Katherine, 18 weeks)

Feelings of similarity with other pregnant women and with women in general became more prevalent. Katherine felt suddenly thrilled by a shared moment with another pregnant woman she did not know. Linda found her new sense of connection with women expressed even in dreams.

> Yesterday a woman in the store asked me how far along I was. I was thrilled. We were both 5 months along. I felt so much like I was sharing something special with her. (Katherine, 22 weeks)

> I dreamt I was at a women's group, sitting in a circle of women. Although I didn't know any of these women, I felt I had much in common with them, and I felt nurtured by being with them. (Linda, 14 weeks)

Social occasions with friends took on added dimensions if young children were included. Women imagined themselves in the maternal role or watched their husbands with an eye to the future as they interacted with the children.

> We went out 2 weeks ago with a couple who have a baby. I watched Bill with the baby. It made me feel good to think of what it will be like to see him with our baby. I've never seen him so attentive to a child. (Katherine, 22 weeks)

More universal feelings of being connected to other people or of moving into a different generation emerged.

> There is this extraordinary, acute awareness of unity with other people that is sometimes overwhelming to me . . . a feeling of real connectedness with other people on a level I haven't felt before. (Anna, 19 weeks)

> knowing you're going to be a parent feels like stepping up the ladder. (Rachael, 24 weeks)

In contrast, adjusting to the new visibility of their pregnancy in the second trimester proved more conflicted in the work environment. Women found themselves more frequently stared at and came to appreciate this attention less and less as pregnancy went on. Feelings of discomfort and even shame at the obvious manifestation of their sexuality emerged in the work sphere.

> People are beginning to react to my pregnancy at work. Other staff members are beginning to greet me with things like "Hello, pregnant lady," and it makes me angry. At times I feel excluded from professional conversations. As soon as I walk up, the conversation stops, then shifts to talk about babies. It makes me feel odd and bizarre. (Rachael, 23 weeks)

> People at work are noticing now. It's funny, but I've had feelings of shame—shame about getting "knocked up," of succumbing to the woman's role and getting ensnared in it. I've felt shame about no longer being really free and a "career woman." (Katherine, 20 weeks)

In time, the women did become somewhat more accustomed to being stared at and treated differentially at work, even though they never really became comfortable with it.

Changes in general psychological orientation in the second trimester were reflected in changing attitudes toward work. By the time Linda felt physically improved enough to return to school and resume part of her studies, for example, she found herself suddenly less interested in the intellectual aspects of the class which had greatly appealed to her earlier. Katherine experienced difficulty concentrating and often felt sleepy during the day, while Rachael found herself more emotionally vulnerable to the ordinary ups and downs of her work day.

At the same time, there were occasions when the structuring and cognitive demands of work could counteract the more affective and mentally disorienting effects of pregnancy. When this occurred, women either felt inhibited in their fantasy life with regard to the pregnancy or simply felt temporarily less connected to the pregnancy altogether.

> I'm feeling deficient in fantasy life. I feel like I'm working all the time and there is no time to think about the pregnancy. (Katherine, 21 weeks)

Rachael mentioned similar feelings. She spoke of the baby "dropping" in her awareness during a particularly busy period at work. Findings by Myra Leifer (1980) suggest that there are links between the quality and intensity of an expectant mother's fantasy life during pregnancy and her evolving relations with her child. Women in this study found that when work intruded too insistently on their attention or dominated their energies for too extended a time, they felt less intimately connected to the pregnancy. This certainly suggests that fantasies and thoughts about the pregnancy are indeed an important aspect of sustaining the developing relation with the fetus. The women who worked throughout the second trimester expressed their shift in attitude as a reordering of priorities in which commitment to the unborn child gained increasing ascendancey over ongoing work concerns.

Thus, the integration of work and motherhood took on more complexity. In addition to the demands of work and the psychological effects of pregnancy, pregnant professional women were now confronted with the emotional significance of their condition for others in their work environment and with their own newly fluctuating priorities. These women's interpersonal worlds during the second trimester became increasingly fluid and complex. Emotional shifts in the marital relationship, in relationships with family and friends, and in the work sphere indicated the extent to which identities were in flux.

The Third Trimester

The third trimester was characterized by renewed closeness in the marital relationship and increased interest in those external conditions specifically related to the pregnancy and to active preparations for the child. Interest in work decreased markedly as libidinal energies became entirely directed towards the events of labor, delivery, and anticipated interaction with the child. Because of their increased size and feelings of vulnerability, women viewed themselves as more susceptible to the environment. Fatigue, restlessness, and other renewed physical symptoms left women feeling less interested in social activity, although this was also the time for baby showers and visits with family. The obvious nature of their condition also produced a loss of anonymity with strangers who felt free to make comments or give unrequested advice.

The critical importance of the marital relationship could be more directly expressed in the third trimester, as women started childbirth classes with their husbands and began organizing the baby's room. Feelings of irritability or conflict with the marital relationship dissipated and more feelings of satisfaction and partnership emerged.

> I feel like some of the strains and the distance I was feeling with my husband before have just seemed to go away. It's not like there was this big thing that we had to resolve; it's just like the strained feelings kind of went away. (Linda, 33 weeks)

> Since the due date's become imminent, he's gotten real busy doing things, building shelves and that kind of thing. It's pulled us—made us feel closer, because I can see that he is really there with me. I'm not just the one having the baby; *we* are pregnant. (Linda, 34 weeks)

At the end of the second trimester, Anna experienced intense anger with her husband because he could not share her experience fully. He seemed less interested than she did in the pregnancy and this left her feeling very alone and disconnected from him. The third trimester, however, started with an important dream in which Anna searched for her husband in a hostile environment, found him, discovered he had amnesia, and carefully set about reestablishing her connection with him.

> My husband and others were committed as adolescents to an orphanage. He had done something wrong, and this was his punishment. I searched for him and found he had been taken to this orphanage. I infiltrated the building. I saw him and saw that he and the others were suffering from some kind of amnesia. He and I had been deeply in love, but he had no recollection of his other life. I got him out, but he still had no memory. I held a pair of shoes I wore a long time ago, hoping to trigger his memory. I felt infinitely patient, an unwinding cord of connection and love. I told him his true name was John. I awoke feeling that joy of refinding him and felt deeply connected and patient with the unfolding of that connection with him. (Anna, 26 weeks)

In the dream, themes of crime and punishment, of parental neglect (the orphanage), and forgetting her (amnesia) neatly combined to give expression to her feelings of anger at her husband's separateness and his inability to fully share her preoccupation with the baby. Yet reconciliatory themes remained the dominant features of this dream. In spite of his unmentionable crime, she looked for her husband out of love and found him, although he had forgotten her. Once she released him, she set about renewing their connection with infinite patience and care. After this dream, Anna felt a vivid sense of restored relationship with her husband. This sense continued to deepen as she began to work with him in natural childbirth classes.

> Seven weeks from now he [the baby] joins us. The birth is real. Now I can only think ahead as far as labor and delivery. I expect it will be hard work physically, but I trust I can do it. I feel much trust and partnership in working with John at the birth. (Anna, 29 weeks)

Like Anna, Katherine, who had previously found her husband less attentive to her than she would have liked, now found that he was being very attentive to her. He helped her with preparations for the child's room and attended birth classes with her. She felt close and trusting of him in a new way. Rachael, who had not felt dissatisfied with her husband's level of involvement, felt even more closely bound to him. She found that she was able to trust him and let herself depend on him in new ways.

> In my childbirth class, I realized I had come a ways in allowing myself to be more dependent on James. Before I felt we were equal, or I took care of him. During the pregnancy I have learned to trust him more about taking care of me. He does things now that are new, like rubbing my back and filling the car with gas. I trust him more to be strong for me. (Rachael, 28 weeks)

The sense of deepened commitment and closeness in the marital relationship experienced in the third trimester brought to fruition earlier feelings of commitment expressed at the time of conception. The feeling of being partners in the transition from childlessness to parenthood which was at times shaken by the crises of pregnancy was now reaffirmed. The imminence of delivery brought the special intimacy of life without children into focus. Thoughts about the impact of the baby on the couple's relationship prompted new appreciation for the marital bond.

> I still want to preserve my relationship with James. I don't want the baby to permeate my whole life. (Rachael, 35 weeks)

Anna and her husband took a special "last" vacation as a couple.

> Our last vacation as a couple was everything I wanted it to be. I felt connected to John as a couple. I feel secure about that connectedness in the triangle that we are to become. (Anna, 33 weeks)

For these women, the marital bond remained central throughout the pregnancy cycle. Beginning with conception, feelings, thoughts, dreams, and fantasies often referred to the marital matrix. The strength of this bond, its adaptability, and its limitations, together with the actual physical and emotional effects of pregnancy, became the groundwork against which women began to work out their individual patterns of motherhood.

Family relationships were also important. All of the women either went to visit their families or had family visit them at home sometime during the third trimester. Interactions with family at this advanced stage of pregnancy could dramatically affect the way women felt about themselves. Rachael described visits with her family and with her in-laws.

> We went to visit James' family. They're down-home sort of people. They were so happy and excited to see me. They felt my stomach and my sisters-in-law were very physical and involved. Everyone was protective of my lifting things. I felt so skinny, healthy, and beautiful! . . . My parents were more reserved, more withdrawn. My mother joked about her "fat, chubby" daughter. Weight makes everybody in my family anxious. I felt like an elephant, so big. (Rachael, 28 weeks)

Katherine, who also went to see her family, found her own sisters very interested in her pregnancy, revealing a mixture of envy and curiosity. Her father was quite attentive, and she felt closer to him. To her surprise, she found herself thinking that she would really enjoy having her father come out and visit after the birth. Until this time, she had been more aware of her feelings for her mother during pregnancy than for her father. Her interaction with her mother remained more ambivalent. She felt disappointed that her mother was not more attentive and began to wonder how much she would be able to depend on her when her mother came out to visit after the birth. The time with her in-laws was marked by feelings of discomfort. Her sister-in-law was unable to have children and had adopted a child. During the visit with her, Katherine's pregnancy was pointedly ignored. Only references to "next year when I see you with your baby" were made. The feelings of discomfort evoked by this visit turned into depression at the next visit with friends. Here, Katherine's pregnant state was in striking contrast to the nonpregnant slenderness of her friends. One of the women even felt "mild disgust" at Katherine's size. For both Katherine and Rachael, family visits were a blend of mixed feelings. Each was made acutely aware of her changed size and shape. Themes of warmth and excitement alternated with themes of rivalry and embarrassment.

Linda and Anna were both visited by their families. Linda's parents and her siblings came out during the summer. She enjoyed the visit, especially with her siblings, but felt less close with her mother than she would have liked. Anna's mother came to visit her at her request. It became very important to Anna to have her mother see her while she was pregnant. Before her mother's arrival, Anna fretted and worried that something would happen to her mother and she would miss seeing Anna pregnant. In fact, her mother arrived without difficulty and they had a rewarding visit. For the first time, Anna felt that she could accept her mother and see her clearly.

> The visit with my mother was good. I so much wanted her to see me pregnant. I feel I am finally able to see my mother as a whole and complete person. I can finally give up my picture of her as less than me. There is somehow no further investment in continuing to feel superior to her. (Anna, 31 weeks)

The change Anna experienced in her relationship with her mother was not felt by other women in this study. These women continued to feel that their relationships with their mothers remained as they had been earlier in pregnancy. Nuances in this relationship introduced in the second trimester did not lead to the dramatic shift experienced by Anna in the third trimester.

It is likely that these women's emphasis on a different definition of the maternal role, with more even division between maternity and professional interests, put them at greater odds with traditional models of childbearing. This dual commitment as well as their decision to delay childbearing itself may have made reconciliation between mothering styles of their generation and their mother's generation more conflicted. However, it should also be noted that academic and professional achievement motivation in women is generally correlated with specific types of affective relationships within the family.

Women oriented toward achievement often report warmer relationships with their fathers than with their mothers (Worell & Worell, 1974). Professional women in this study did, in fact, see their fathers as the more nurturing figure in their background. While the specifically female nature of pregnancy led all the women in this study to reflect on their relationships with their mothers, only one of them experienced a significant shift in her perception of her mother at this stage. The other women reported only minor shifts.

The importance of relationships with friends for support and a sense of community gained in significance in the third trimester. Baby showers or dinners for the expectant parents were events of special warmth and meaning.

> Friends gave us a baby shower that was really nice. It made me feel like there was a community of people around who already care about the baby and who will be there for us. (Rachael, 31 weeks)

Role rehearsal with children of friends or relatives continued to be a source of confidence and pleasure. All of the women now talked about feeling confident that they would be able to mother their children.

In contrast to the importance of relationships in their private lives, work and work relationships meant less and less. Only two of the women worked during part of the third trimester. In general, they found themselves less able to concentrate or invest their energies in what they were doing. Katherine felt irritated with people who kept her waiting or seemed to be wasting her time. Rachael, on the other hand, felt like she wanted to avoid conflicts. She found herself becoming very accepting of things she would normally have resisted.

> I can tell sometimes when my patients are doing something to manipulate me. But I just don't care. I feel like I just want to "be" with my clients. I want to value and appreciate them or hold them on my lap and cuddle them. (Rachael, 34 weeks)

Feelings of fatigue and exhaustion added to the sense that work was becoming not only less interesting but also physically overwhelming. For Katherine, who was less professionally developed than Rachael, these realities underlining the complexity of integrating work and motherhood proved more anxiety-provoking. She wondered how she was going to be able to finish her dissertation or keep working after the baby arrived. Her experimentation with the reality of integrating work and motherhood was reflected in the way she arranged her house. In the second trimester she had insisted on putting her desk and the baby's crib in the same room. She imagined being able to study in this room while pregnant and perhaps even after the child arrived. What she found in the second trimester was that she spent her time in this room looking at the crib and daydreaming while she actually worked in other parts of the house. In the third trimester, she made a clear separation between her work space and her mothering space.

> I am moving my desk to the second bedroom. I've decided to have the baby by itself. It's been hard to work in this room. (Katherine, 34 weeks)

Yet her decision to move her things felt unsettling. She had to keep reminding herself that the room would soon be filled by the baby. Several weeks later, after the birth of the child, she found that the time she had planned to spend studying when her child was sleeping was taken up by household chores or simply resting herself. The frustrating aspects of integrating work and maternity which she experienced during pregnancy continued after delivery and remained a long-term project.

Their increased size and the obvious nature of their condition made these women the object of comments and advice from strangers at work and on the streets. The comments were experienced as personal and intrusive, although the women tried to make light of them. Katherine talked about a young man whom she didn't know coming up to her at work and making pointed remarks about how she must be married. Linda said she had people approaching her in the street during the last month of her pregnancy and advising her to go home because she looked ready to deliver at any moment.

In the last weeks of pregnancy, women felt little interest in anything but the impending labor and delivery. Career interests, friends, family, everything faded into the background except thoughts of childbirth and feelings of security in the marital relationship.

> I feel supported by John. I am really able to get it, his support. I feel I can count on it in labor and delivery. (Anna, 34 weeks)

> There will be other people around when I give birth, but he [my husband] will be the mainstay. (Katherine, 36 weeks)

The renewal of closeness felt in the early part of the third trimester was consolidated into a feeling of trust and security in the marital relationship by the end of the third trimester.

Relationships in the third trimester were centered around issues of preparation for the baby's arrival and the consolidation of earlier emotional commitment. In the marital relationship, this took the form of feeling more connected and certain of the husband's dependability. Active preparations for the baby and working together in natural childbirth classes deepened feelings of partnership and mutual participation in the pregnancy. Awareness of the impending shift from a dyadic to a triadic family constellation made the last weeks as a couple a time of special closeness. Visits with family took on symbolic significance as couples prepared to become parents and parents to become grandparents. The importance of friends and social networks during this time lay in their ability to provide women with support, interest, and a sense of community. Friends who already had children became important role referents. Playing with or caring for friends' children gave women an opportunity to practice role rehearsal in anticipation of interacting with their own child.

The reordering of priorities with regard to work and motherhood in the second trimester shifted more completely in the direction of motherhood during the third trimester. Women still perceived work as rewarding and did not abandon long-term professional goals, but they felt less and less inclined to pursue current work interests. Their emotional energies were dominated by the immediacy of labor, delivery, and impending motherhood.

Labor and Delivery

Relationships during labor and delivery were necessarily limited and narrowly focused. All of the women had their husbands present throughout labor and delivery. Three women had friends present as well. These relationships and those with the attending midwife or medical staff followed a similar structure. The relationship with the husband remained emotionally primary and central, while the relationships with medical staff were more functional. Only when husbands or friends left did relationships with medical staff assume great emotional significance. The presence of friends was supportive but emotionally more peripheral.

All of the women had prepared for childbirth with their husbands and hoped to deliver in alternative birth centers or, in Katherine's case, at home. Although all three women who delivered in a hospital needed special medical intervention, husbands were not barred from the delivery room and were able to stay with their wives during labor. Without exception, women felt that the presence of their husbands was critical to their emotional well-being at this time:

> I really knew that my husband was absolutely supportive of me and would be a strength to me in labor. I really counted on that, too; that was vital to me, to know that I had a partner and that I could trust him and rely on him to work with me. (Anna, labor and delivery)

Besides symbolizing strength in addition to her own strength, Anna saw her husband's presence acting as a counterpoise to her fears of the unknown. His ability to play this role was enhanced by virtue of his being a doctor himself, but Anna emphasized the stabilizing influence of his emotional significance as compared to his medical knowledge. She did not rely on him to make medical decisions but turned to him as an emotional focus throughout her long and exhausting labor.

Similar feelings about the husband's role during labor were voiced by Katherine and Rachael. Rachael's reaction to a break in her husband's emotional availability simply underscored this point:

> When I would be awake and unable to sleep for contractions and James would be asleep, I would feel very angry and alone and abandoned. It wouldn't make sense for him to stay up for 48 hours, so it was a good thing he was getting some sleep; but at the time I was angry and hurt and felt very alone. (Rachael, labor and delivery)

In the absence of her husband, she relied more heavily on nursing staff. She described her labor nurses as very sympathetic and supportive, helping her in "all kinds of ways."

For two women, emotional support and practical help with breathing and relaxation techniques were extended by friends who acted as auxiliary birth coaches. Katherine, who delivered at home, had various friends offering encouragement and support in relays throughout her labor, while her husband and her midwife remained the principal birth coaches. Not surprisingly, women friends asked to be present at the birth as coaches were already mothers themselves. Almost all of the women attending the birth at Katherine's house were mothers, too. No doubt the presence of other women who had experienced labor and delivery was reassuring. Katherine's feelings that she would "die" if she didn't somehow endure the painful intensity of what she was experiencing bear witness to the sense of extremity which can accompany labor and delivery.

Linda, who did not experience labor because she had a planned C-section, found the presence of her husband and her friends as emotionally important as the other women. The impact of unpleasant standard hospital procedures was given a humorous twist as she acted out her fears for her friends, although the degree of medical control necessitated by her type of delivery was particularly distressing to her. Like Rachael, she commented on the importance of a supportive nursing staff:

> It was a matter of sitting in one of the delivery rooms and getting all the—getting the IV, the enema, shaving the pubic hair, and all this stuff you don't do when you're going to an alternative birth center. I really didn't like it . . . having a C-section clearly means the medical staff is in control. I didn't like it, but fortunately, I had very, very nice nurses and I sat there with no clothes on, with my huge belly sticking out. One of my friends took a picture of me grimacing . . . And there were the doctors and then I got on the table . . . So I lay there—I heard my friends outside the door . . . The idea that I was lying there, and that all my friends were out there, just moved me so much so I was crying. (Linda, labor and delivery)

Although her husband could not help her with labor, his presence in the delivery room provided the same support and stabilizing influence that other women experienced.

> My husband was sitting by my head, holding my hand; and we were just looking at each other with those kinds of unspoken but very—well, they were very profound looks. (Linda, labor and delivery)

Delivery itself, experienced with excitement, relief, and wonder, was a special time for husbands and wives. For these women the awe of having produced a child, of holding the baby at last, was seconded only by the joy of sharing the moment with the baby's father:

> I heard a baby cry . . . and we both were crying . . . to be sharing that together and hearing her cry. This whole next 10 minutes were part of that special moment. (Linda, labor and delivery)

The sense of partnership and having worked well together through a difficult time could even lead to feelings of euphoria:

> I just was flying, and so in love with this baby and so in love with my husband. (Rachael, labor and delivery)

Once delivery was over, three of the women were able to share the excitement and feeling of celebration with friends. Anna, who delivered at the hospital where her husband worked, received a steady stream of visitors and well-wishers. Linda talked and joked with friends. Katherine, surrounded by her women friends, now joined by some of their husbands, celebrated with a real birthday cake and champagne!

The patterning of relationships around labor and delivery was quite similar for these women, regardless of the type of delivery they had. Husbands became a primary source of strength and emotional focus during labor and delivery. Their presence was highly valued and felt to be a stabilizing influence in the emotionally charged surroundings of a medical hospital. Friends, as birth coaches or as a more peripheral source of support, were viewed as adding an important dimension to the childbirth experience in terms of community or shared celebration. Obstetricians and other medical staff played a vital but emotionally secondary role in labor and delivery, unless the husband was unavailable. In the husband's absence, the support of medical staff became crucial. The emotional tenor of interactions with hospital staff was vividly remembered. Small acts of kindness or indifference were experienced with considerable intensity when women described their hospital stays. The absence of mothers during the time of childbirth was remarkable, considering the importance of their presence in more traditional models for the birth of a first child. Only one woman had her parents come out close to the time she was due to deliver. The other women waited until they had settled into their new mothering roles before inviting mothers to visit.

Postpartum

Predictably enough, the main focus of women's lives after childbirth was the child. The desire to hold and be physically close to the infant was profound:

I was just awed by this amazing process of physical birth, and that here at the end—
I thought that was the end then—here's this person. And I just wanted to go over that
person all the time and the only way I could relate to it was "hands-on." It was very
physical . . . all I wanted to do was touch him. I don't have words for that time. They
were very animal feelings. (Anna, postpartum)

The need for physical closeness was satisfied by holding the infant, sometimes for hours on end, and by the special union of the nursing relationship. This delicate and vulnerable relationship was extraordinarily
significant emotionally. Outside influences as well as the actual flow of
interactions or "fit" between mother and child could seriously affect its
satisfactory unfolding. Women reported feeling intense joy when feedings
went well and distress or despair when they did not. Two women, in
particular, felt literally traumatized by environmental events which intruded into the nursing relationship, in each case with what women felt
were negative and long-lasting results. While still in the recovery room,
for example, a nurse had tried to "help" Anna start the nursing relationship with what seemed to Anna a lack of sensitivity to the delicacy of the
relationship being initiated.

She [the nurse] just took his head and pressed his head onto my nipple and I remember
this moment feeling so raped . . . My feelings were outrage for myself and for him,
that we weren't given the support to learn how to do this in more "Let him do it at
his own pace." And I felt for both of us and I felt I needed somebody else to help us;
I felt so vulnerable, I really felt so vulnerable I couldn't take care of myself. (Anna,
postpartum)

Eventually, Anna did establish a satisfactory nursing routine with her
child. Yet she continued to feel that nursing would have gone much better
if she had been given more supportive nursing instructions. She added
that her difficulties in nursing had left her feeling badly about herself in
relation to her child. In contrast to her difficulties with nursing, other
postpartum discomforts that were the result of the delivery itself, such as
the episiotomy, did not cause her particular emotional distress.

Like Anna, Linda had difficulty establishing nursing. In her case
there were even more external referents. The baby's pediatricians, her
mother-in-law, and even friends became involved in ways that left her
increasingly anxious and uncertain of herself.

Then we started this thing about nursing, which proved very difficult. It was a real
hard time for us. My breasts weren't the kind which were easy for her to glom onto
. . . and evidently she was not a good sucker. So even though biologically what happened with my body was pretty normal, we had a difficult time with nursing, because
she just wasn't interested. I got very worried about it. I was so uptight that I wasn't

aware of the letdown reflex. The letdown is when the baby sucks enough to bring the back milk down, which is the richer milk. Plus I had my mother-in-law standing over me, and I had all these doctors insisting that I come in and show them I had milk in my breasts. It was horrible, and I got more and more uptight. I felt bad. I felt I had failed her [my baby]. . . . Then I had friends who'd call and say, "You should nurse her on demand." (Linda, postpartum)

Linda, like Anna, eventually worked out a satisfying feeding routine with her child, mostly through patient efforts and by gradually becoming more aware of her own and her baby's rhythms.

The sense of having a "family" of one's own with the increased responsibilities of caring for a child led to changes in the marital relationship. The women felt a deepened commitment to the marriage and developed new respect for their husbands as fathers:

It's really changed my relationship with my husband, deepening it in a lot of ways. It makes me feel like there is a unique connection with him that I hope never to have with anyone else, of having created this life together and having joined in some kind of amazing union. I feel very safe with him and very trusting of our partnership and very respectful of the way he fathers and the way he is with her. (Rachael, postpartum)

At the same time, the loss of privacy and the demands of childcare created a sense of distance within the marital relationship:

how much it demands of one to give to a child takes away a lot of our energy for one another. On the day-to-day surface of things, we've probably become more distant. We have less time to intensely talk with one another. We're more tired. There's often a child there with us who has her own demands and her own needs and keeps us operating in the present and not talking about some of the things that we're thinking or feeling on a nonmundane level. (Rachael, postpartum)

Three of the women found themselves assuming more stereotypical mothering roles. Anna had anticipated this. The other two women became more conflicted about this change as they tried to resume their academic plans. Suddenly the complexity of mothering and continuing career activities became very real. The difficulty of finding reliable and good infant care was considered a major problem. These mothers found it took a long time, approximately a year in fact, to fully return to their previous career involvement. Only Rachael managed to integrate her personal and professional worlds without major difficulty. She was able to take maternity leave from her job, return to her work on a part-time basis, and share all the early infant care with her husband, who also worked half-time.

Relationships with mothers also changed. As the women saw their mothers with their own children, they were reminded of warm moments they themselves had spent with her as children. The nuances in their relationship with her that began to emerge in the second trimester, and that were integrated for Anna in the third, now crystallized for other women as well. At times they found themselves reevaluating their views of their mothers in a more sympathetic light.

> It was after my baby's birth that the first really positive memories of my mother emerged. After the baby's birth I also went out and bought myself some clothes to return to work in that were more like the kind of clothes that my mother would've liked to have seen me working in all these years. It seemed like I was not only having more positive feelings about myself, but also about her. I remembered more of the things she did give me when I saw her with my daughter and saw how loving and giving she is with her. (Rachael, postpartum)

Summary

These findings illustrate some of the complexities introduced into a woman's interpersonal world during a first pregnancy and after the birth of her child. Changes in the marital relationship, in relationships with family and friends, as well as the integration of personal and professional concerns, occurred in interaction with the physiological and psychological effects of pregnancy. Individual responses varied, but the overall pattern that emerged in the couple relationship was one of confirmation, differentiation, resolution, and consolidation. The first trimester was experienced as a confirmation of the couple relationship, although new concerns about the husband as a potential father also emerged. These new concerns, together with increased awareness of gender differences, led to greater differentiation within the couples' relationship during the second trimester. Women felt more in tune with universal aspects of female experience and were generally closer to their women friends. Feelings of anger or distance in the marital relationship were especially common at the end of the fifth and the beginning of the sixth month of pregnancy. The differentiation experienced as a result of these events was resolved as the couple worked together to prepare for labor and delivery. After the birth of the child, both confirmation of the couple in terms of deepened commitment and differentiation in terms of the distance introduced by the child's presence into the marital dynamic were consolidated into a richer, more complex relationship.

Other changes with family and friends also moved in the direction of complexity. Women perceived themselves as dissimilar from their mothers early in pregnancy but introduced nuances into these views by middle or late pregnancy. Finally, they integrated their feelings of dissimilarity with their new perceptions and achieved a position that allowed them both to appreciate their mothers and view themselves as different from them. Relationships with friends were primarily a source of ongoing support throughout the pregnancy. Friendships with women, especially women who already had children themselves, become more important as pregnancy progressed. Thus, pregnancy placed a woman's interpersonal contacts in a different context. Increased affiliative needs for support, attention, and acceptance made women more dependent on their social networks to maintain their satisfaction with the pregnancy.

Both the physical and the psychological effects of pregnancy interfered with professional and academic plans in the integration of work and maternity. Nausea, fatigue, and the gradual reorientation of psychological focus and libidinal energies made intellectual concentration draining and eventually less appealing altogether. Interactions with colleagues were frequently ambivalent as pregnancy progressed. Only one woman in this study was able to integrate her personal and professional worlds fully, within a few months of giving birth, due to the optimum conditions of her situation.

The last three chapters have presented findings with regard to these women's overall experience of the physical, psychological, and psychosocial effects of pregnancy. But the experience of pregnancy is also an event that occurs in the specific context of an individual's life. The next chapter will discuss each of these women separately and examine the individual themes they evolved to integrate their experience of having a first child.

7

Individual Differences: Developmental Themes in Pregnancy

Overview

The reproductive urge, while biologically motivated toward the preservation of the species, is nonetheless initiated and experienced by the individual woman within the context of her own history and development. Women in this study often became aware of the universal aspects of their experience, but also constellated their experience around themes of particular importance to them. These predominant themes served integrative, organizing functions. They reflected specific developmental issues that varied from woman to woman. This chapter will look at these themes and examine the individual maturational or integrating principle at work in each woman's experience of her first pregnancy.

The themes presented evolved naturally as each woman reflected on her experience from week to week. In this way, developmental themes emerged or were built up during the process of reflection itself rather than being derived from formal history taking. Each woman introduced developmental themes in response to her particular life situation. The woman introduced these themes early in pregnancy and returned to them again and again as the pregnancy progressed. Particular insights, dreams, and events connected to the pregnancy were interpreted in light of these themes until an overarching sense of the pregnancy as a whole began to emerge.

Anna: Motherhood as Individuation and Autonomy

In her thoughts about becoming a mother, conception and pregnancy were already linked to developmental issues in Anna's mind. With reference to conception, Anna spoke of first needing to develop herself in her relationship with her husband. She saw this development as something that depended on her ability to define and reveal herself in their relationship.

This demanded that she "open new sides of herself" and "grow up" in her relationship with her husband. She defined these efforts as "symbiotic unhooking" and "doing this myself." These issues of separation-individuation and autonomy remained central issues for her throughout each stage of the maternity cycle.

Anna described herself as having "come together" with her husband around age 19. During this phase of early adulthood, their relationship included several separations and reunions. Her understanding of these years, which include the period Levinson (1978) has called the "Early Adult Transition," was that she and her husband "grew up together." The growing up together was an extension of Anna's need to share life with a close companion or "twin-like" figure. The pattern for this type of relationship was set in childhood when Anna developed an exceptionally close relationship with her brother to insulate herself from feelings of loneliness or solitude. Her early years with her husband recapitulated this pattern and helped to support her transition into early adulthood. This transition was further consolidated by marriage in her mid-20s.

Anna's need for closeness as a way of defining herself was also reflected in her relationships with friends. She described herself as having several very close women friends with whom she also felt she had a "symbiotic" relationship. What she meant by the term "symbiotic" had to do with the way she used these relationships to define her sense of self. By focusing on the other person in such a relationship, Anna avoided an independent definition of self.

> I think when you're symbiotically hooked up with somebody else—that's my experience, at least—there's a diffusion of awareness. I just don't have to be aware of what's going on inside me, because I can just turn it all on the other person, whoever the other half is. Growing up seems to me to be knowing I'm not going to be twins with anybody. That I am really on my own. (Postpartum)

In this way, Anna's relationships were the source of much shared life experience and were fundamentally based on mutual empathy.

The one area where her life differed from that of her friends, however, was in childbearing. Her friends had already had children in their 20s, while she delayed starting a family until she was 31. While her relationship style had given her the support she needed in her 20s, it had left her less certain of her ability to do things on her own. Despite her educational training, she felt that she had not found her life work and had actually stopped working a few years before she had her baby. When Anna felt she was ready to conceive, she first experienced her sense of readiness passively as a "willingness to cooperate" with whatever being it was she felt making contact with her and wanting to be born through her. This feeling was immediately followed, however, by the intuition that having a baby would also require some active preparation on her part. She formulated this as needing to "grow up" in her relationship with her husband and "doing this [the pregnancy] alone." She had felt his support and sharing as they "grew up together," now she wanted to discover her capacity to support herself and make her support available to her child who would necessarily be dependent on her. In this way, Anna's pregnancy became a vehicle for separation from a previous style of relationship and individuation into a more autonomous sense of self.

The initial changes of pregnancy, the sense of separateness and growing internal preoccupation mentioned by all the women in the first trimester, were experienced by Anna as increased awareness that she could not share her pregnancy in the same way that she had shared other things in her life. Her own sure sense that she was pregnant even before medical confirmation, for example, was not shared by her husband. She realized more concretely than before that he could not feel what she felt when he became prey to anxieties about the reality of pregnancy that she did not experience:

And John doesn't have the inner sense of trust that I feel because he isn't in me. So this has started the theme for me around this pregnancy that "Nobody's sharing this with me; nobody knows this or feels the things I feel and I can't make somebody feel what I feel." It's been painful. (5 weeks)

Similar feelings of emotional discontinuity also emerged in her relationship with her best friend. Anna found herself becoming angry that her friend was not as involved as she wanted her to be.

Began to feel furious with [friend] that we couldn't be there [in the "vast wilderness" that symbolized feelings of loneliness for Anna] together, hand in hand. She can't go with me or help me bridge the gap. I'm up against myself here, no symbiotic twinning will help me through it. This is mine which I must do. (5 weeks)

At the same time she realized that it was now necessary to redefine the closeness in her relationships to allow for a more individuated identity, both in relation to others and in relation to her expected child.

I'm working with [friend] to untie the symbiotic knot I have with her toward my being separate now and also to avoid this state with my child in the future with he or she. (5 weeks)

When she expressed some of these feelings to her husband, he offered his support and wondered if he "could be there" with her in the way she needed. His response was in keeping with their established relationship style. Even in early pregnancy, however, Anna found that she could not accept his offer unequivocally. She felt instead that her present feelings of separation made his offer "too much to contemplate."

[My husband] mentioned, could he be there? For now it's too much to contemplate. I just don't know what to do. I just feel nobody can do this with me. (5 weeks)

The verbal skills which Anna had turned to in the past to articulate her feelings and bridge the distance between herself and others no longer seemed adequate to communicate the nature of her experience in pregnancy. The intensification of internal imagery in the form of dreams and fantasy life appeared to her as "levels of perception" for which there was "no verbal or even cognitive translation." For Anna, these changes were critical factors in modifying subtle aspects of her psychological orientation while leaving more global personality characteristics intact. It is important to note that these changes, while profoundly felt subjectively, did not disturb her overall behavior which remained adequate and organized.

While a sense of separateness and gradual withdrawal from external concerns produced mild depressive feelings in Anna, it was especially the "loneliness" of being pregnant that impressed her. This loneliness peaked at two different points during the pregnancy—once just before the appearance of the first fetal movements and once shortly before delivery.

The first peak in feelings of loneliness, at 16 weeks, was perceived more diffusely than the second. "I feel lonely. The loneliness is different from depression. I don't know what it is exactly." At the time, Anna wondered if her feelings were stimulated by developmental processes. "I considered the possibility of individuation. Could separateness cause these feelings of loneliness?" The question remained unanswered for her at this point, however, because not long after Anna felt her baby move. Her awareness of the fetal movements occurred the same night she dreamed that the baby showed itself to her. In the dream Anna was being examined by a nurse practitioner when suddenly "my belly rose up like a whale and the baby showed himself to me." She interpreted the dream as a sign of affection and communication from her unborn child; therefore, feeling her child move had a great effect on her prior feelings of loneliness. She now felt supported by the continually felt presence of her baby in her womb. The fetal movements allowed her to feel merged with her child. The fetus became her "partner" in the pregnancy, initially dissipating her feelings of loneliness. While she still felt separate from others, her baby held out the possibility of a new symbiotic attachment. It seemed like an ideal partnership, and Anna felt many feelings of satisfaction and well-being during the second trimester of her pregnancy as a result.

Gradually, however, it dawned on Anna that she was the adult in this partnership. Whereas before she had depended on "symbiotic" relationships to support her, this relationship was one in which she was the support for another during a critical life transition. She was the one who would take the initiative and provide active maternal support to her baby. The realization of her maternal responsibility renewed some of her feelings of loneliness, but it also promoted feelings of autonomy.

> I am feeling alone in the sense that I am the only one who can give birth. The same with being a mother. This is the reality. It's the way it is. I am not fearful and feel I can do this. (24 weeks)

Thus, the reversal of the original mother-child symbiosis was first experienced fully by Anna only in the context of her first pregnancy. The experience was a powerful one, reminding Anna of earlier efforts toward individuation in her life.

The second peak in feelings of loneliness occurred one weekend in the third trimester, a few weeks before delivery. Once again, Anna felt overwhelmed by feelings of loneliness and responsibility for her fetus. She became desperate in the absence of her husband and her close friends who were all temporarily unavailable to comfort her. With no one she could turn to to assuage her distress, she was forced to deal with her loneliness by herself. In the process she had an important moment of insight during which all her feelings of loneliness suddenly crystallized into a new perspective on herself.

> I was terribly alone, desperately lonely. As the day wore on, I knew that there was something useful for me to see. The theme of my pregnancy, the alone thing, became focused, pinpointed. It was that I am alone, no one can do anything to alter that. I got through that aloneness and realized that nothing from the outside can make me whole. I am whole. (33 weeks)

The realization that she had a center within herself from which to act was a developmental step for Anna. Previously she had relied upon her relationships with others to supply her with a sense of direction and "wholeness" in life. Now she found that she did not need outside reassurance in the same way.

This insight also had another important outcome. It allowed Anna to develop a different perspective on her relationship with her child. Because she was more in touch with her own purposefulness and autonomy, separate from her husband and her friends, she also became clearer about the nature of her relationship with her unborn child. When she became clearer about the boundaries between herself and others, she also became clearer about the boundaries between herself and her child. She knew, for example, that she would care for her infant, but now she also realized that he would bring distinct characteristics and predispositions into the world with him that she could neither predict nor assume total responsibility for. Her more realistic appraisal of the situation modulated her earlier anxieties about the responsibility of motherhood and allowed her to feel her baby's prospective independence from her. Perceiving one's baby as a locus of being and of feeling independent from oneself is just as important an aspect of healthy mothering as tolerating the baby's developmental need for a more merged identity. This is so because the mother's perception of her baby as a person in his/her own right both mirrors and facilitates the development of mother-child mutuality.

After childbirth, Anna continued to integrate these developmental gains with regard to individuation and autonomy. She continued to view herself from the vantage point she had attained during her pregnancy. This new perspective emphasized her greater psychological independence from others.

> I do feel—I know where my life comes from in a way I didn't know before. I mean I know it comes from me. Nobody else is gonna fill in the blanks. And that's a basic point of view which changes everything. (Postpartum)

Given Anna's inclination to structure her relationships in terms of "symbiotic" needs, she was well-prepared to identify or fuse with her baby *in utero* and after birth. She was less well-equipped to view herself in the active mothering role and see her baby as separate from herself. Consequently, much of the work of pregnancy for Anna constellated around developmental issues of autonomy and individuation. Throughout the pregnancy, she interpreted different aspects of her experience in light of these issues. The extent to which the content of her anxieties about "symbiotic unhooking" and "doing this myself" accurately pinpointed and subsequently focused on the areas in her development she needed to strengthen is quite striking. This may be an example of the power of innate drives directed toward growth and maturation, which many writers (e.g., Erikson, 1959; A. Freud, 1965) assume to be a part of basic human developmental processes. In any case, Anna's experience does suggest that a first pregnancy may bring into focus and help integrate specific issues significant for ongoing development in adult life. In her case the central importance of these issues of autonomy and individuation grew out of her previous life experience during which she had built up life structures that emphasized needs for affiliation over needs for autonomy.

Rachael: Motherhood as Dependency and the Integration of Personal and Professional Worlds

Rachael's pregnancy raised different developmental issues for her than those Anna experienced; but like Anna, Rachael also linked together the notion of personal development and childbearing. For her these issues centered around dependency and the integration of her personal and professional worlds. In contrast to Anna, Rachael had consolidated her professional identity and her work world. She had established her autonomy and felt comfortable being self-reliant and independent. Becoming pregnant was symbolic of this stability in her life and her marriage. For Rachael, it was the developmental issues raised by her feelings of dependency during pregnancy and the complexities of integrating her professional identity with her identity as a mother that formed the basis of her pregnancy experience.

Throughout her 20s, Rachael's initial life structure in early adulthood included a series of provisional personal and work arrangements. She described herself as having had "three main [love] relationships in life," as well as a progressively more defined commitment to professional life. During these years, the areas of love and work seemed to move in tandem with each other, until they culminated in full commitment to both marriage and profession by age 30. The decision to have a child was symbolic of this established sense of direction in her life.

The idea of having a child evolved slowly within the framework of Rachael's love and work arrangements. She graduated from college and married her first husband in the same year. They married "without discussing children" and "later we fought about the issue." Her husband was not interested in having children. During her marriage, Rachael continued to take courses at a local university while she held various jobs unrelated to any specific professional commitment. Eventually she decided to go to medical school. After her first year, she divorced and lived for a time with a man she described as "passionate, exciting, and a great lover" although he was also "moody, unpredictable, and we often argued." Already unhappy in the relationship, Rachael finally left when her lover told her that he also was not interested in being a father and probably was infertile anyway since he had failed to have children in his two previous marriages. As she finished her third year of medical school and this relationship ended, Rachael realized that part of her attraction to the men in her life had been based on their ability to make her "feel safe." They were further along in age and professional development, and she had relied on them to provide her with a sense of security. Now she no longer needed this kind of protection. At this point she met her second husband, whom she liked because he was "gentle and kind." They lived together for several years while she finished medical school and her internship and residency. They married when they decided to conceive a child together.

Rachael's life experience in her 20s reflected a pattern of experimentation with various ways of combining love and work. She managed her uncertainty about adding motherhood to this combination by choosing men who were not interested in becoming fathers, thus deferring all but the discussion of childbearing issues. Only when her professional identity was assured and her love relationship secure did she attempt this more complex integration. Her dual commitment to family and professional life manifested itself in the fluctuating balance of interest between the two at different times during her pregnancy. This balance of interest had two distinct poles, each representing mutually exclusive self-concepts with opposing characteristics:

> During this pregnancy I've had to accept and incorporate sides of me which I've crowded into little corners and didn't like so much, didn't value so much about me. I mean I was identified with my more active, logical, out-there-in-the-world, skinny— all these things go together for me—independence, not-needing-anybody sides of me. That's what I had really tried to be and stress. And I can be none of those things too well, since I've become pregnant. (23 weeks)

Her soft, vulnerable, more dependent side was the side she identified with motherhood. While she could visualize herself in the active mothering role, Rachael had real resistance to accepting the more passive, yielding aspects of gestation and nurturing in which the mother lends herself first to the needs of her developing fetus and then puts herself at the disposal of her newborn infant. She formulated her awareness of this resistance to the increased dependency of pregnancy in terms of questions about her maternal capacities:

> I have recognized feelings that run as a theme throughout the pregnancy for me, of wondering am I gonna be able to nurture and take good enough care of this life, and is this me, am I cut out for this? (20 weeks)

To counteract her anxieties about becoming more dependent in the early months of pregnancy, Rachael threw herself into her professional life with added fervor. She accepted additional responsibilities and even took on some teaching assignments and speaking engagements. She struggled to maintain her usual level of energy and involvement with external concerns. At this point she interpreted the intensification of her internal imagery, which occurred in the form of erotic dreams and fantasies about her athletic prowess, as "wishful thinking" or due to the influence of hormonal changes. It was not until sometime in the fifth month of her pregnancy that she started having dreams in which she found her concerns so clearly symbolized that they drew attention to the profound transformation she was experiencing. She spontaneously began to work through aspects of the dream material and discovered that it helped her to integrate her experience. An example of such a dream and her interpretation of it follows:

(The Dream)

> In this dream I was roaming around inside these large houses; actually, whatever the large building was kept changing its form. At one time it would be a house; at another time it would be a college dormitory; then other times it would be more like a museum. And I was roaming around through them and felt very lost and disoriented about where I was. I knew I had to get from the top floor of the structure into the basement; and it was very difficult to find my way and to get there. I kept being afraid, as I was going through, that I was somehow going to lose my purse. Someone was going to take it from me, or I was gonna mislay it or lose it in some way. And later in the dream, as I was getting lower and lower in the structure, it turned out I had lost something. I'd lost a shoe. And I couldn't leave the house without it. As I looked for it, I kept catching sight of myself in mirrors and seeing that my body was really huge and distorted-looking.

Rachael's interpretation of the dream:

> When I think back about the dream and what it seems to be saying, everything seems so rich to me. That I am lost is how I think I am beginning to feel, that my old self is lost in so many ways. That my body is lost, that my old sense of identity is getting lost. And I am feeling in a huger body than I am used to, and I am also feeling—as in the symbol of the dormitory—I am feeling a loss of privacy is ahead of me. And having to share with people and be in a tighter space than I am used to being. And the idea of losing my shoe—I mean both of those I associate with competence in the world and having my valuables about me and being able to get around and be independent and take off and go where I want to go. Those things I am losing, too, as I am getting tied down into a responsible relationship with an infant. So even the idea of going from the top floor into the basement seems a lot like what this pregnancy has been like for me, of going from my head and my intellect, my thinking/functioning part of me through this kind of regression that I really experience as what this pregnancy's about, to rock-bottom somehow, to the basement and the unconscious, I guess. Somehow that home part of me, the vulnerable, passive, dependent part of me—the basement represents that part of me, getting down to something very at the bottom of things. (22 weeks)

It is clear from her interpretation that Rachael viewed becoming a mother as a "regressive" process, compelling her to lay aside her intellect and independence and taking her back to sides of herself she had held in abeyance or categorically suppressed during her 20s. The level of her accomplishment and self-definition in a culture which traditionally discourages such development in women had not been easily won. By the time she became pregnant, she had spent years working to integrate her work life with a settled love relationship. She had defined herself in this relationship as "just kind of having everything under control myself and not needing much from him [my husband]." Pregnancy altered this self-reliant self-image. After the birth of her child, she described her experience of becoming more dependent quite clearly.

> I felt like the pregnancy was a whole process of getting a little more passive, a little more regressed, and for a while fighting that and feeling negatively about myself and then coming to accept it. And then as soon as I would accept it, I would get a little more that way and get negative about it again, and then have to accept it more. And—till by the end I was just completely self-absorbed and hedonistic and wanting to sit around and do nothing and didn't want to work any more, and just wanted to nest and be taken care of. And it—it was a long road to get there. (Postpartum)

Her negative feelings about her increasing passivity during pregnancy acted as a stimulus. She became preoccupied with the problem of integrating her images of herself as a professional woman and a mother. She recognized that she was attempting to readjust internal images she had built up as issues from earlier developmental periods emerged. As she gained weight, for example, she recalled her adolescent problems with weight and reexperienced her fears of "being fat" and out of control. The emotional dichotomies she had created as she pursued her professional development were conflicted. Home signified dependence, vulnerability, and constraint, but also warmth, security, and love. Professional life offered self-definition and autonomy, but suppressed her "homey" sides. The process of reassessing and integrating these images occurred gradually throughout Rachael's pregnancy.

At work she found herself reacting angrily to what she felt was her colleagues' view of her as a "walking uterus" and felt protective of her professional status. At the same time she found her interest in work declining once she met the extra work commitments she had assumed in the early months of pregnancy. She experienced tension between her external professional concerns and the internal preoccupation reported by all the women in this study as a feature of pregnancy. It was hard to know whether to struggle against the passivity she felt or to give in and, in her mind, risk losing the developmental gains of her 20s. Ultimately, she did allow herself to depend more on her husband and to curtail work and social activities. In the process she discovered new strengths in her husband and new respect for his fathering and nurturing abilities. She also gave more expression to the "homey" sides of herself.

But this change did not come about without anxiety. Like the other women in this study, she sometimes felt isolated by virtue of being pregnant, surprised by the intensity and rapidity with which pregnancy began to affect her life, and caught between the conflicting pressures of impending motherhood. She was in her seventh month when she had a dream which directly addressed her anxieties:

> I had a dream that I'd had the baby and was forgetting the baby for hours at a time because I was so busy with my work. During one of the times that I had forgotten about the baby's existence and was working on other things, the baby began to sort of fade away and become transparent. When I remembered that the baby existed again, my baby was almost a perfectly clear, glass kind of infant. In a panic, I remembered the baby was there and I put the baby to my breast and just sort of watched this milk pour into the baby, who was transparent at that point. It was like pouring milk into a glass. As the milk filled the baby, the baby started to get its color back again and to be alive and okay. (28 weeks)

On reflection, she found the dream reassuring, a sign that she would be able to resolve her situation and be able to provide the necessary care for her infant:

> This dream seems like it's definitely expressing how hard it is for me to think of myself putting together my work life and my mothering. I just don't know if I will have the energy or time to give to both and make them go well. The other part of the dream seems like a positive statement about the fact that I will be able to take care of a child, to give it life and sustain it. (28 weeks)

After the baby was born, Rachael found that moments of transition between work and mothering proved the most difficult. It was always hard to leave her baby and go to work, though she was happy to be at work once she arrived. It should be reiterated here that Rachael had an unusually supportive situation with respect to infant care. She was able to take three months' maternity leave from her job. After that, she and her husband shared child care. They each worked half-time and looked after their daughter half-time. This freed Rachael to continue developing both sides of herself. She was pleased to discover that "I am a good mother and I'm able to do it real well and have a lot of nurturing and love inside me." She found that her ability to mother gave her a new perspective on her work.

> In some very deep way I feel more confident of myself now than I ever did before becoming a mother. I feel like I really know I'm good at this and it's the most important thing, even more than whatever my professional success might be. It puts the ambiguities and insecurities of the profession in balance for me to say I know I can mother and I'm happy with this part of my life. (Postpartum)

Her work on integrating her professional and maternal identities by coming to terms with her needs for self-reliance and her needs to be taken care of was reflected in a more flexible self-image which allowed her fuller emotional expression:

> I think I have felt permanently more vulnerable and more responsible and more emotional. I'm less defensive in my feelings than I was before. I still find myself crying over a lot of things that really touch me that would never have brought tears in earlier days. I feel a different sense of respect and connection to all mothers and fathers in the world, a sense of community I didn't experience before. (Postpartum)

Rachael stressed the development of independence and competence in her first adult life structure. She defined herself professionally as a doctor and interpersonally as a partner in a committed love relationship. The experience of her first pregnancy after she turned 30 brought out the submerged sides of herself. While Anna needed to develop more autonomy during her first pregnancy, Rachael was faced with the task of acknowledging her dependency needs. Her anxieties constellated around "losing control" and what it meant to become dependent on her husband. Again, it is striking how the content of her anxieties was developmentally focused; that is to say, her anxieties highlighted precisely those rejected aspects of herself she needed to incorporate. Like Anna, becoming a mother stimulated Rachael to make this incorporation which resulted in a more integrated perspective on herself and her life.

Katherine: Motherhood as Initiation into Female Adult Identity

Anna and Rachael presented developmental themes in pregnancy which can be considered complementary in character. They focused on facets of their personalities they had previously neglected and worked to remedy the unevenness in their development which had been the result. Katherine's developmental themes took a somewhat different form. They were structured in terms of initiation rather than complementarity. For her, becoming a mother was primarily associated with issues specifically related to feminity in adulthood. These issues became central themes throughout her pregnancy, integrating earlier developmental concerns and defining areas of growth. At various times she described her progression through the different stages of the maternity cycle as a process of initiation into "a community of women."

The importance and developmental significance of communal female experience found its origins in Katherine's personal history. One of three sisters, she remembered special feelings of connectedness with her siblings in childhood. These feelings motivated her to seek out friendships with women and stimulated her interest in women's issues later in life. They shaped themes of rivalry and competition when they arose, although the general tenor of Katherine's relationships with women was one of valued fellowship and shared experience.

After Katherine graduated from college at 21, she worked in a community agency where she met her husband. Her job ended several months after they met. Without further employment or funds, she decided to look for work in another city rather than stay where she was and risk becoming dependent on her future husband who was then her boyfriend. "Our relationship was not at that point yet," she said. While separated for the next seven months, they maintained contact and visited each other frequently. After this separation, they both found jobs in another state. They moved there together and lived together for a year before they married. Katherine was 23.

They lived in this state another 2 years. It was during this time that Katherine joined a women's consciousness-raising group where she found a "wonderful connection with a group of women." Some of these women were mothers, but she had "no connection with them around their kids." Prior to her own pregnancy, Katherine described herself as one of those women "who would have ignored a pregnant woman" because she would have felt vaguely threatened by her condition, "fearful of this happening to me." It was also during these years that Katherine began to define her professional interests and met her first female role model in the profession.

At 25, Katherine and her husband moved again. This time Katherine was unable to find work in her area of interest without having a graduate degree. Although her professional interests were more defined, she delayed starting graduate study at this time. Instead, she didn't work but took courses at a university to define her interests further. When she was certain of her direction, she asked her husband to move for her sake so she could start graduate school in another state.

The move marked a turning point in her relationship with her husband. Her husband was more than 10 years her senior. More mature and professionally more advanced than Katherine, he had played a mentorial role for her in the early years of their relationship. Now she found he could no longer play that role. Her field of study demanded different skills than his, and her new interests introduced her to an intellectual orientation that was unfamiliar to him. As she began to reformulate her own experience in terms of what she was learning, she also reviewed her idealized view of her husband and began to see him more clearly. She said her desire for a child was connected to her loss of this idealized image. She had the "feeling I was grown up. . . . I finally felt adult enough to have a child."

Katherine's 20's were largely structured by her relationship with her husband. He defined where they lived, and many of his ideas provided the context in which they articulated their social and political interests. Although her close relationships were not "symbiotic" but cooperative or mentorial in style, Katherine's life structure during these years, like Anna's, was predominantly colored by affiliative needs. At the same time she defined her professional interests and began altering her first life structure to reflect these interests as she approached age 30. She decided to become pregnant once her studies were established and experienced becoming a mother as symbolic of her adult female status.

The emphasis on "adult female" grew out of earlier developmental concerns related to her physical development in adolescence. At the time she developed more slowly than her peers and didn't start menarche until 16. This had her worried "whether I would ever get to be a woman." When she became pregnant, she immediately felt "very womanly." As her breasts started to swell, she remarked that she felt like she was "going through puberty" and felt happy that "my body will finally become a woman's body." In Katherine's mind pregnancy symbolized the full expression of her female sexuality, finally banishing any remaining questions about her essential femininity.

Despite the discomfort they could cause, Katherine greeted the physical changes of pregnancy as welcome indications of her satisfactory progress. She experienced the changes as linking her to other women.

I feel similar to other pregnant women. I feel a sense of relationship with them even though I don't look very pregnant yet. (17 weeks)

Like Rachael, who, when she first felt fetal movements, summed up her feelings about her pregnancy with the telling phrase, "I feel like I'm doing a good job," Katherine responded to the same experience with the equally revealing remark, "I feel I'm developing like I should." Both phrases captured an essential aspect of each woman's orientation to her experience.

The other women in this study also mentioned their increased feelings of closeness to women in general, and to women with children in particular, generated by their pregnancy. To various extents, all of them felt that pregnancy gave them a new position in the life cycle, but it was

Katherine who formulated this change in terms of a specifically female experience with ritual dimensions. Communicating her sense of the special bond between women created by their shared experience as childbearers, she first used the phrase "community of women" in the second trimester to describe this feeling.

> I spent the weekend with a friend who saved her maternity clothes and offered to let me use some. I feel like I'm moving into a community of women, sharing a universal experience—the kind of thing all women go through. (21 weeks)

The feeling of being in touch with a primordial aspect of female experience remained central throughout her pregnancy and after the birth of her child.

The sense of being connected to other women, first felt toward her sisters in childhood, had reemerged in her 20s when she joined a women's consciousness-raising group. Now pregnancy added another dimension. Just as the women she had encountered earlier provided her with a "wonderful sense of connection" at the level of her emerging identity as a young adult, so now she became part of an expectant mothers' group as she began to develop her maternal identity. She remembered the earlier group in terms of her efforts to define herself and explore her emerging professional interests. This group focused on childbirth techniques and exchanged information about the vicissitudes of pregnancy and early infant care.

This group of women also became a source of emotional support and "community" in the face of her unsatisfactory relationship with her own mother. Already in the first month of her pregnancy, Katherine had called her mother with the hope she would be able to "connect with her around this pregnancy." As described in chapter 6, this proved a difficult and frustrating experience. Katherine's mother was unable to provide what Katherine wanted in the way of a role model or to act as a source of information. Still, many of her thoughts during pregnancy were preoccupied with her mother and the kind of mothering Katherine had received from her as a child. Her memories presented a mixed picture. She remembered warm family meals but also her mother's preference for another sibling.

Perhaps it was these associations which formed the underlying context in which themes of rivalry with other women began to emerge. First Katherine talked about her disappointment that her mother refused to sew maternity clothes for her even though she frequently sewed clothes for her sister. Then she spoke of her sister's mixed feelings of "envy and curiosity" about her pregnancy. Finally, she mentioned her own feelings of envy toward a pregnant friend.

> Despite feeling awful [physically], one of the strange feelings I had was very strong envy when I went to the flea market with my friend. She is pregnant and almost full term. At the market we were getting a lot of attention, but she was getting more— more than me, and I felt envious. (29 weeks)

Themes of envy and rivalry may also be considered to represent more primitive emotions of particular significance in relation to pregnancy because they bring to light the underside of female solidarity expressed in Katherine's image of a "community of women." While women are linked by the universals of feminine experience, they are also rivals in the sexual and reproductive drama. Feelings along these lines emerged in near archetypal form in one of Katherine's dreams early in the third trimester.

> I had delivered the baby in the hospital. It was the day after, and I hadn't seen it yet. I went into the nursery with two friends. One of them immediately picked up the baby and sat and nursed it! I was very upset and anxious. *I* wanted to hold the baby. *She* shouldn't be holding it. *I* should be. After her, the other friend took the baby. I was so distraught and frantic, just touching the baby all over. (27 weeks)

The themes in this dream are structurally reminiscent of similar themes in fairy tales. In these stories the natural mother is, in one way or another, deprived of her child by the machinations of one or more jealous female rivals. Usually the depriving figures are an older witch or wicked fairy, a figure with maternal characteristics resonant with oedipal themes. But there are other stories even closer to Katherine's dream. In these, like the story of Solomon confronted by two women each claiming to be the mother of the same child, the depriving figure is a peer.

In her dream, Katherine's situation is less extreme, but she is nonetheless temporarily deprived of her baby by another woman. The fear of losing one's child or having it taken over or stolen by an envious woman is a very primitive one. It arouses much anxiety and provides the rationale for many of the charms and rituals used to protect parturient women in preliterate societies. Contemporary psychological thinking locates the origin of this anxiety in deep-lying levels of the personality, stemming from the earliest rivalrous feelings experienced toward the mother (Breen, 1975). Given Katherine's closeness with other women and her reliance on them for support during her pregnancy, it was not surprising that her feelings of rivalry and envy emerged in synchrony with her more positive conscious attitudes.

Katherine's earlier worries about her delayed physical development in adolescence naturally predisposed her to anxiety-laden comparisons between her own feminine development and that of other women. During her first pregnancy, she both reached out to other women in search of role models and felt rivalrous toward them with respect to her still-developing maternal identity. Her approach to her own mother replicated these feelings. She longed for more maternal support and felt rivalrous with her preferred sibling. Eventually, Katherine began to sort out these feelings. She gave up her efforts to be close with her mother; she came to terms with the mothering she herself had received and began to work out the mothering role she planned to adopt vis-a-vis her own child.

Katherine's overall pregnancy experience affirmed her sense of adult female identity. It organized itself around issues predominantly related to a change in status. The changed status was developmentally focused with respect to Katherine's personal history. While Anna and Rachael experienced submerged sides of themselves emerging in their experience of first pregnancy, Katherine's experience constellated around specifically feminine psychosexual issues. Her experience more closely resembled the structure found in traditional *rites de passage*. For her, the sense of separateness and the intensification of internal imagery, felt by all the women in this study, may be loosely compared to the isolation of the initiate and the visionary experience most often associated with initiation rites typically found in many early cultures. Here, too, the rites entail tests of endurance and physical pain, followed by full acceptance into the adult community. Two weeks before delivery, Katherine had a dream which psychically replicates this structure:

> I was set off on an island with Nazi guards. I wondered if they would abuse me. Later I saw a woman who was going off to have her baby. I wanted to watch to see "how it was done" on this island. She was wearing a long white gown and sat on a white horse, preparing to ride off to an isolated part of the island. I became this woman. My time came. I had a white bird with me, giving me strength and companionship through labor. When the labor was over, the bird looked tired. I looked upon it with gratitude. Then I slept with the baby next to me. I woke and knew I had to leave. The bird changed into a cat. I understood it was my only protection. Later it changed into a rabbit. I got on the horse and returned to my living quarters. When I arrived, my women friends ushered me into a room. Excitedly and immediately they wanted to see how I looked after delivery. I took off my clothes, revealing a flatter stomach but also a deep fold of skin. Someone asked if I felt a loss. I did. (35 weeks)

In the dream Katherine finds herself on an unknown island with frightening aspects to it. She is then preceded by another woman who "shows her the way." She retreats to an isolated part of the island and gives birth, surrounded by archetypal symbols of female fertility—the bird, the cat, and the rabbit (Neumann, 1955). Then she returns to her "women friends"—a community of women—and shows off her body to reveal the marks of her initiation ordeal. The gesture is accompanied by a feeling of loss which gives expression to the mourning inevitably attached to the passing from one state to another. After the birth of her child, Katherine did, in fact, experience sadness over the loss of her single, more carefree days.

Once she became a mother, Katherine's feelings about having entered a new stage in the life cycle solidified. She perceived her old self as "rather frivolous and selfcentered," responsible only for herself "like a child." Now she felt older. She used the image of the "matriarch" to describe her feelings.

> Once you have a child—at delivery—you step into a territory where you will never be untied. It's made me feel merged with others. All women feel like sisters now, in terms of that bond [having a baby]. I guess the word "matriarch" comes to mind. I feel matriarchal in the sense that I am concerned with others and watching over them. It has to do with wisdom and being an adult rather than a child. (Postpartum)

Katherine spent her 20s consolidating her relationship with her husband and slowly defining her professional interests. She stressed first her commitment to her marriage, developing a more individuated sense of herself within that framework. Then she began to define her field of interest outside the marriage. Having a baby was connected to a series of transitions in her life. She lost her idealized image of her husband, settled on her profession, and started a new course of study during the transition from her 20s to her 30s. She added the transition into motherhood at the same time. Undergoing so many important changes at once may have amplified her sense of ritual passage from one state to another. While she experienced pregnancy colored by earlier developmental issues, as did Anna and Rachael, themes of initiation rather than complementarity predominated. In the end, she too developed a new perspective on herself which incorporated earlier concerns and promoted a fuller sense of herself.

Linda: Motherhood as Conflict

The discussion of Linda's pregnancy experience with reference to issues in adult development is complicated by her special problems during this time. Her experience was unusual in terms of its physical intensity and generally debilitating effects. Her struggle to cope with these physical discomforts and the emotional conflict they aroused became the central dynamic of her pregnancy. She did express a number of the same universal themes mentioned by the other women in this study, but these remained largely overshadowed by the conflict which marked her overall experience. Linda's experience raises a number of questions. Not all can be answered, but her perception of her experience does present valuable information about how a woman feels when her pregnancy is traumatic.

Linda's condition, known technically as hyperemesis gravidarum, consisted of excessive vomiting—an exacerbation of the morning sickness commonly experienced by women in early pregnancy. Psychoanalytic theory associates this problem with unconscious rejection of the child and/or rejection of the female biological role. It considers hyperemesis a psychosomatic response to negative psychological factors. The medical view finds hyperemesis a rare condition whose exact cause is not yet firmly established but which is generally connected with a multiple pregnancy, a hydatidiform mole, or the result of some hidden infection, especially in the urinary tract (Bourne, 1972). In fact, psychiatric treatment of this condition has not been very effective, and it is presently treated by medication or, in cases of dehydration resulting from excessive loss of fluid due to vomiting, by hospitalization. Psychiatric treatment is usually sought only for treatment of previously existing psychiatric disorders (Bourne, 1972). The following discussion does not attempt to resolve the lack of consensus between medical and psychoanalytic views, nor does it presume to give a definitive account of Linda's experience. It does present her view of the matter and her feelings as she struggled to deal with her situation. It also offers some tentative interpretations, based on an interactionist view of development which takes into account the reciprocal influence between an individual's psychology and the social context in which this psychology is played out (Thomas & Chess, 1980).

Like Katherine, Linda finished college when she was 21. After graduation, she made her first attempt to leave home. She was "pinned" to a fraternity man, so she decided to move to a city close to the town where he lived. There she found work and set up house by herself. In her mind she was "doing the prescribed thing—go to college and find a man to marry." But her relationship with this man proved to be "a disaster." Alone and away from home, she became more emotionally dependent on him than he could tolerate and the relationship broke up. Linda returned home feeling "devastated." She remained home for almost two years, first recuperating from her love affair, then working with much success and enjoyment as an assistant manager for a business concern. Gradually she realized that "life was extremely comfortable at home" and that she could "spend my life there and never do anything." This realization precipitated her second move away from home.

She moved further away than the previous time and set up house with her old college roommate, with whose help the decision to move had been made. She felt fortunate this time because she met "an older man" who "took care" of her during the first year she lived in her new home. He helped her find work and showed her the way around. Linda enjoyed the relationship but did not think of it in terms of a long-range commitment. "He didn't fit my image of who I was supposed to be with." He was 15 years older than her and of different ethnic origin. He was also unable to have children due to a vasectomy. When she was 25, Linda broke off this relationship to pursue a relationship with a man her own age who more closely resembled her internalized image of what a potential mate should be. The relationship was "sexually passionate" but unstable—"on again, off again," in her words. The relationship lasted a few years but never developed into the committed relationship she wanted. By age 29, she felt she "had to make a change." This prompted a third move.

This time she moved to the west coast by herself. She had "no job, no money, and only the apartment of a friend to stay in." Until she found full-time employment she worked at a series of "horrible" temporary jobs. It was a difficult time. She did resume a friendship with an older woman she had known earlier in her life. This woman was more liberal in her views than Linda's parents and had "always turned me on to things I found helpful." Now this woman suggested that Linda participate in a study and problem-solving group. Linda joined this group and it proved to be a turning point in her life. It was here that Linda began to define her views and develop a political focus. She was attracted to feminist philosophy and discovered a point of view which seemed to summarize much of her experience in the world up to that point. It was also in this setting that she met her future husband. She was 31 years old.

Although they were part of the same study group, it was not until the group ended that Linda and her future husband began going out together. She remembered thinking, at the time, "I could take this man seriously." Still, she found it difficult to "relax and believe that this was what I'd been looking for all these years." The first six months of their relationship were problematic. He was not willing to state his commitment to the relationship and Linda "tested him about everything." Eventually she began to insist on some more defined commitment in the relationship. It was another turning point for Linda. "I really grew up and took myself seriously in this relationship. I asked for what I wanted and decided that I would have to be met in terms of what I needed or I didn't want the relationship. I was no longer afraid to be alone." Instead of feeling "so emotional," she started to feel a new sense of strength and self-appreciation. Her demands provoked a brief separation but eventually led to a reconciliation and a firm commitment on his part to their relationship.

After this they lived together for another year and then married when Linda was 33.

This was also the period in which Linda began to take herself seriously with regard to her professional interests. An older couple who had been supportive during the time she and her husband had been deciding about their relationship took her aside one day and said, "You really have to do something with your life. What is it going to be?" Their challenge brought the issue of her professional development into focus. With their encouragement, she started graduate school and found she "loved it" and was good at her work.

By the time she was 35, she felt she was ready to have a child. Her marriage was settled and she had now established her professional direction. She talked with her husband about it and the decision to have a baby was mutual. She carefully worked out the timing of her pregnancy to coordinate with her academic schedule and felt pleased when conception was confirmed.

From Linda's early adult history, it is clear that she experienced initial difficulty in accomplishing the developmental tasks of that time. Despite her drive and motivation toward independence, the larger pattern of Linda's 20s reflects much conflict and uncertainty and little focus. She had trouble leaving home and was unsuccessful in her attempts to establish a long-term love relationship. She did not develop specific interests or define career goals, although she was a reliable and even talented employee. It seems fair to say that Linda was caught between her conflicting needs for dependence and autonomy. She wanted independence but was unable to establish herself on her own without considerable external support. She was good at her work but did not think in terms of defining her professional interests or upgrading her skills. Instead, she tried to follow the "prescribed" pattern of college and marriage. When this failed, she continued to structure her life in ways that proved unsuccessful in resolving the conflict. At 29, she was alone, with neither a love relationship nor a sense of professional direction. It was at this point that she felt she "had to make a change."

In evaluating Linda's early adult history it must be remembered that her difficulties in meeting the developmental tasks of this period can be seen not only in terms of her personal psychology, but also as a reflection of her position in history. Caught in the crosscurrents of the conflicting social values of her generation, she had internalized both the traditional feminine pattern of "college, marriage, and motherhood" as well as the emerging pattern of feminine independence stressed by the women's movement. From this perspective, it can be hypothesized that the interaction between her personal dynamics and her social situation no doubt reinforced her conflicts. Unfortunately, this was not advantageous to Linda. It amplified her conflict around issues of dependence and autonomy and made their resolution more troubled.

For these reasons, it is not surprising that much of the conflict generated by the severe physical problems she experienced during her first pregnancy constellated around precisely these issues. While she had made a number of changes in her first life structure during the transition into her 30s, these maturational gains were perhaps not yet well enough consolidated to withstand the extra strain imposed by her physical condition during pregnancy.

When Linda became pregnant, she had no way of predicting how she would feel. Not unlike many people, she had assumed that her life would continue pretty much as usual during the time of her pregnancy. In her mind she thought she wouldn't be doing anything particularly active: She would be gestating. Within a few weeks of conception, however, she started feeling nauseated. This was not especially anxiety-provoking. She knew many women experienced nausea in early pregnancy. But in her case the nausea kept increasing until it became the dominant feature of her life.

> I've been having a rough time. I feel very sick and tired. I've had to drastically cut back my schedule of outside commitments and now spend much of my time at home. It's hard to keep food down and I end up in bed most of the morning. I feel so overwhelmed by it right now it's hard to believe it will stop. (9 weeks)

As her own experience continued to diverge from the "storybook example" and even from that of other pregnant women she knew, Linda began to feel more and more isolated. She felt angry that no one had warned her about this "darker side of pregnancy" and frustrated by the dramatic impact her symptoms exercised over her life. She found she could not leave the house without a paper bag in case she needed to vomit unexpectedly. She could not eat meals with her husband because the smell of food made her ill. She lost weight and felt weak with hunger, though she couldn't keep anything down. She was worried about the medication she was taking to help counteract the nausea because new research suggested that there might be harmful effects to the fetus from this medication. There seemed to be no relief in sight. She was just "surviving from day to day."

The dimensions of her physical distress were paralleled by emotional effects. She was alternately angry, depressed, and self-critical. She felt more and more responsible for what was happening to her. "I had a lot of people saying to me during the pregnancy that my attitude had something to do with it, or my resistance or my ambivalence. From Linda's perspective, how could anyone not be ambivalent, considering the nature of her experience?

> I feel like every woman has ambivalence when they're pregnant. I mean your body is being invaded and there are ways that, when you say that—that your body is being invaded, that your whole being is being intruded upon—that sounds hostile. But it's not necessarily hostile. Sometimes I feel real hostile about it, but sometimes I don't. I just feel like it's a fact, and I feel like, "Why don't people understand the psychological changes around that? Why don't people understand the impact on your life when you're going through that?" (Postpartum)

The interpenetration of self and other is a powerful experience in pregnancy. It profoundly alters the boundaries that define ordinary existence. The sense of fluidity introduced into the personality during pregnancy by the emotional lability and increased internal preoccupation that are regular features of the experience puts stress on a woman's psychological economy. A degree of physical discomfort in the first trimester may help concretize this process and support a woman's sense of reality about the pregnancy. When physical symptoms so override manageable limits, however, the stress itself becomes the object of preoccupation and interferes with the woman's ability to maintain her self-esteem or sense of mastery over the situation. This is what happened to Linda. She lost all sense of "a future" and simply tried to manage from day to day.

> I'm so damned fed up. Today was a better day, in terms of nausea; but tonight's bad and what have I got to look forward to? I just hang in day by day, TV all day, nothing different, everything lousy. No guarantee of change. I'm so damned angry and depressed I can't even cry. My life feels like shit. I hate it. (12 weeks)

When the first trimester ended and brought no relief—morning sickness in pregnancy generally occurs only in the first trimester—Linda's anger and depression turned to despair. She had thoughts of suicide and abortion as she contemplated spending the rest of the pregnancy struggling with her nausea. At this point she became so dehydrated from loss of body fluids by vomiting that she was hospitalized. In the hospital she was put on IV fluids and given medication for her nausea. Gradually the symptoms subsided and Linda regained a sense of optimism.

> The biggest thing I remember about that was just the joy that I could actually eat a normal meal and keep it down and not feel sick. I remember sitting there in that bed in that hospital, thinking "I feel like a queen. I could never feel any better. Nothing could make me happier than how I feel right now, because I have been taken care of.

They did something to me that made me feel better and I got to eat something."
(14 weeks)

She was in the hospital a few days and returned home greatly improved.

This hospital stay was followed by two other events, amniocentesis and, a few weeks later, the appearance of fetal movements. These events together with her continued physical improvement, marked the turning point of Linda's pregnancy. Now the baby inside her, rather than her physical distress, could become the focus of her preoccupation. The amniocentesis also revealed the sex of her child. Since Linda and her husband wanted a girl, the news increased Linda's satisfaction with her pregnancy. She continued to have feelings of being "invaded" physically by her fetus, but these feelings did not inhibit her sense of being attached to her unborn child. She began to wonder about her child and looked forward to seeing it after birth. The fetal movements helped her feel more personally in communication with her baby as she learned to distinguish different types of movements and came to recognize specific patterns. By the last trimester she even began to experience the "bloom of pregnancy" she had so often heard about.

A strictly psychodynamic interpretation of Linda's experience would most likely focus on her unconscious conflict about having a baby and the unresolved oral needs of her childhood. Such an interpretation would no doubt hold some truth. But in the case of such a psychobiological event as pregnancy it may also be helpful to look beyond the specifics of individual psychology. Speaking from a broader theoretical perspective, Simone de Beauvoir (1952) suggests that a woman's development of her individuality inevitably brings her into conflict with her role as preserver of the species in childbearing. A woman's instinctual side is thus, to some extent already, intrinsically at odds with her individuality. De Beauvoir argues that it is this built-in internal dilemma which is manifested in women's greater number of physical ailments related to their reproductive system. She interprets these ailments as symbolic of the revolt of the organism against the subordination of its individuality to survival of the species. She writes:

> The more clearly the female appears as a separate individual, the more imperiously the continuity of life asserts itself against her separateness . . . Woman, like man, is her body but her body is something other than herself . . . Woman [in pregnancy] experiences a more profound alienation [from herself] when fertilization has occurred. It [pregnancy] is often associated in the first month with loss of appetite and vomiting, which are not found in any female domesticated animal and which signalize the revolt of the organism against the invading species. (1952, pp. 25, 33)

De Beauvoir's arguments bring to mind Linda's feelings as she watched her academic plans collapse under the impact of her pregnancy experience.

> And because of how sick I was, I had to drop out of classes, and I still have some incompletes and I never finished my thesis. So that was really a horrible thing for me; because school was a wonderful thing. I loved being in school. I was doing fine, I was doing wonderfully well. And so when I got pregnant, I was just devastated that here was this wreck in my plan and that it was a plan that I was enjoying so much. (Postpartum)

From the perspective of Linda's early adult history, it seems that it took her a long time to develop an independent sense of herself. She experienced this sense of herself coming together around the changes she made in her life during her age 30 transition. By her early 30s, she had come to terms with the developmental issues of her 20s that had proved so difficult for her. She established herself independently when she first moved to the west coast. She found interpersonal commitment and satisfaction in her marriage and found a professional focus for her intellectual interests. It was a lot to accomplish in a relatively short period. Life felt more settled after these changes, and Linda felt ready to become pregnant.

Her physical illness in pregnancy was unexpected. It made the transition into motherhood severely taxing and struck at the foundation of the second life structure she had just started to develop. For her, having a baby in some sense symbolized the fruition of her earlier efforts—the completion of one cycle and the start of another. The difficulty of the experience upset the balance she had only recently attained. It deferred her professional development, renewing anxieties about her abilities. As her condition worsened, it also impaired the equality she valued in her relationship with her husband, thus threatening her feelings of autonomy.

> One of the worst things that I felt was that I felt an increased sense of dependency on my husband, emotional dependency, physical dependency, and I did not like it at all. It just did not feel good. (Postpartum)

Finally, her distress shook her sense of femininity. In Linda's mind having babies was something that women simply did, "like falling off a log." Her own situation left her feeling vulnerable on all fronts and her sense of self-esteem plummeted. She even began to feel uncertain of her skills as a parent.

When things did start to improve, Linda's self-esteem also improved. In the latter part of the pregnancy, she felt special because she was pregnant and began to enjoy the extra attention and caring of friends and family. She did have to cope with further difficulties. She was unable to deliver vaginally and she had trouble working out a satisfactory nursing relationship at the start. But in the end she did establish a warm relationship with her child and slowly picked up her studies again. Still, her memories about her pregnancy experience were conflicted. She rejoiced in her child, but remained keenly aware of the sacrifices bearing her had involved. She summed up her experience as being both a sacrifice and an affirmation.

> I love my child and having her is something I get a lot from. I get to be part of a family and I like being part of a family. Still, there is sadness in the sacrifice. I feel sad for that part of me that is sacrificed in order to have a child. The affirmation is in having the child and caring for it. (Postpartum)

Linda's first life structure created difficulty meeting the demands of early adulthood. She made various attempts to establish her independence and find a committed love relationship, but achieved only partial success in her efforts. She remained professionally and interpersonally conflicted. It was not until she entered the transition into her 30s that she began to rapidly and successfully rectify the flaws in her earlier life structure. Her second life structure included motherhood. The exact cause of her difficulties during pregnancy cannot be demonstrated, but it can be said that the intensity of her distress interfered with the consolidation of her recently achieved maturational gains. It is possible that the threatened loss of these newly acquired and highly valued aspects of herself not only contributed to, but actually amplified the level of conflict Linda experienced during pregnancy. In any case, it is clear that her incapacitating symptoms marred the experience of becoming a mother. In her mind, pregnancy became a sacrifice rendered worthwhile only by the sense of self-affirmation she felt when actually caring for her child.

Summary

From the preceding discussion, it is obvious that the individual developmental themes emphasized by each woman were to some degree present in all the protocols. The emergence of individual patterns is thus sketched against the overall groundwork of gestation. Other authors (Benedek, 1959; Bibring, 1959; Deutsch, 1944; Kestenberg, 1975) have already argued in favor of the developmental nature of a first pregnancy and have stressed the uniform features of the experience. The individual patterns which emerge out of the symbolic meaning given by the individual to general features of the pregnancy experience are less well-known. This chapter has attempted to understand the particular structure developed by each parturient woman during her first pregnancy in order to clarify some of these patterns. It has also explored the relationship between these patterns and ongoing issues in adult development.

The next chapter concludes this study and presents questions for future research.

8

Conclusions

Overview

This chapter gathers together various observations made throughout this study and discusses them in light of their larger implications. After a brief summary, issues relevant to the way pregnancy has been conceptualized are taken up and some preliminary links with feminine psychology are made. Suggestions for practical applications of the insights growing out of this study are also proposed and areas in need of further research are pointed out.

Retrospective Summary with Some Theoretical Reflections

The introduction to this study argued in favor of investigating women's subjective experience of a first pregnancy in the early 30s to better understand those aspects of becoming a mother that women themselves judge to be important. Such an investigation offers new insights into the nature of this experience and the way women perceive its developmental influence in their adult life. In addition, the perceptions of these women provides information important for a more thorough evaluation of the role of a first pregnancy in the integration of female psychology.

Chapters 4 through 6 presented the overall typology of a first pregnancy as it was experienced by the four women in this study. They also outlined the individual developmental themes each of the women evolved during the course of this experience. The dynamic interaction between general features of the pregnancy experience and the interpretation of these features by each woman along developmental lines was further explored to reveal the underlying structural patterns of complementarity, initiation, and conflict. These patterns may be considered to reflect the organizational structuring of experience by each of the women in this study, a structuring of experience which integrates the effects of physiological, psychological, and societal forces into a synthetic whole. Together, these results contribute to a conceptual understanding of maternity which is directed toward a more comprehensive or "holistic" theory about the specifically feminine experience of pregnancy and parturition.

A review of the general features of a first pregnancy demonstrates that women in their 30s who are expecting their first child experience this period primarily as a time of psychological reorientation. Rapid physiological changes accompanied by equally profound psychological ones lead to the intensification of internal imagery, the emotional lability, and the internal preoccupation which are the psychic hallmarks of the pregnancy experience. These introduce a new fluidity into the balance of a woman's intrapsychic economy reflected in the emergence of repressed material from earlier developmental periods and a more fragile sense of self.

The frequent association between pregnancy and feelings of vulnerability or increased dependency bears emphasis because it appears as a central dynamic in all of the protocols. Regardless of the individual variation apparent in any comparison of developmental themes from one protocol to the next, for example, it is obvious that each of the women in this study felt herself to be more vulnerable and dependent on her surroundings during pregnancy and just after giving birth than at any other time in adult life. Some of these feelings obviously stem from a realistic concern about the potential for physical distress which can occur during pregnancy. Kestenberg (1975), however, suggests that in order to fully understand the particular vulnerability of the pregnant woman and new mother, it is important to consider the childhood and adolescent antecedents of what she calls the "adult inner-genital phase" exemplified by pregnancy. She describes how the regressive behavior in the 2½-year-old little girl generally comes in response to her confusion over feelings that arise inside her and excite her, but which yield no visible product as do bowels and bladder. Kestenberg believes that these "inner-genital sensations" are externalized by the little girl and projected into her fantasy life by the creation of an imaginary baby. Use of this fantasy is reflected in doll play or in the child's assertion that she "has a baby in her belly." For the little girl, the imaginary baby functions as a defense against feelings of confusion or helplessness and relieves internal genital tension. It further serves to help her organize her nonverbal ideas about making babies by eating, defecating, or urinating.

At this early age, the little girl's fantasy baby is not yet well-distinguished from a real baby. It is not until around the age of 3½ or 4 that the little girl becomes quite sure that her imaginary baby is not as good as a real one. Kestenberg claims that this discovery leaves the little girl feeling "worthless, deprived and ugly." A buffer to these feelings, however, arises from the hope and reassurance that she will have babies when she grows up. According to Kestenberg, in adolescence both before and after the advent of menarche, the wish for a real baby recurs with great intensity (perhaps one of the reasons for the near epidemic prevalence of teenage pregnancies in this country and many others.) In our present culture, the young girl typically has to repress the wish for a real baby and postpone it in favor of societal goals that discourage childbearing in adolescence. As in childhood, this adolescent postponement of having a real baby is once again linked to feelings of tension, disappointment, and doubt about one's capacity to produce and care for a real child. These are the reasons Kestenberg gives for the feelings of disappointment, unreality, and unfulfilled wishes which are reactivated in women during pregnancy. She sees these feelings as the source of women's vulnerability at this time.

Kestenberg's ideas are useful in discussing the results of this study because they shed light on the experience of pregnancy as an integrating force in female psychology. Her reasoning, for example, explains the association between having a baby and acquiring an enhanced sense of maturity mentioned by all the women in this study. All of them felt that becoming a mother, at some profound level, involved becoming more adult. This was so in spite of their choice to delay childbearing until their 30s when their adult identities were already fairly well-defined. Indeed, it is striking that, given their level of education and accomplishment, these women still felt that having a child added a more mature dimension to their adult identities than had existed before. They also felt that it was specifically the experience of pregnancy and childbirth which was tied to this change. According to Kestenberg, this could not be otherwise. Only having a real baby would, in fact, be able to make up for the feelings of disappointment and renunciation experienced at earlier developmental stages.

For these reasons having a real baby may also be considered a psychological springboard for generating a more sophisticated integration of overall self-representations. In childhood, the little girl organizes her confusing inner-genital sensations by evolving the fantasy of the imaginary baby. For her, the feelings inside her must mean that she has a baby in her belly. Later, awareness of the imaginary nature of her baby occasions a shift from grandiose fantasy to more tangible forms of play with dolls or other substitute objects. Together, these events contribute to better structural representations of reality. She is a little girl who cannot have a baby in her belly, but who will have one there some day. Her internal genital sensations are reorganized to reflect both her present incapacity to have a child and her future hope of having one.

In adolescence, new and once-again confusing internal genital sensations are aroused in the experience of menarche. These, like pregnancy, are accompanied by physical changes and emotional lability. Restabilizing their disorganizing impact on the personality requires further integration. The changes are organized with reference to the progression of specifically feminine stages of psychosexual development. Menstruation heralds the potential for a real baby. With this possibility in hand, the young girl experiences a strong urge to externalize her adolescent confusion about the changes occurring in her body by having a real baby. A baby would demonstrate her sexual maturity and allow her to organize her identity and her feelings around her child. Deferring pregnancy at this age is linked with sublimation, the pursuit of culturally valued external as opposed to instinctual goals.

In childhood the fantasy of having a baby is exposed by the little girl's physical inability to bear a child. In adolescence, cultural values intervene to support the postponement of the satisfaction of having a real baby. Both stages involve efforts to integrate internal bodily sensations by externalizing and projecting them in more accessible symbolic form. It is the imaginary baby, the toy substitute, and the adolescent's preoccupation with her body which are the "product" of these inner-genital sensations. Throughout development each of these stages contributes to the elaboration of a more complex self-image. From this perspective, attempts at integration can be seen as developmentally focused, that is to say, directed toward the organization of an increasingly complex and differentiated representation of the self. This, of course, depends on the individual's ability to evolve increasingly accurate mental representations of the internal as well as the external characteristics seen as belonging to the self.

In this way, the regressive behavior and confusion caused by the lack of a visible product for internal genital sensations, such as those produced by the bowel or bladder for other internal sensations in the pelvis, mobilize what may be seen as progressive tendencies oriented toward "making sense" of the confusion. The symbolic importance of having a baby thus originates at different levels of development and plays an integrating role in the psychological economy of the growing girl. Nevertheless, the notion of having a baby which emerges as an organizing motif for internal genital sensations in early childhood and adolescence also evokes the feelings of vulnerability and disappointment experienced in response to not having had a real baby before. As a result, the feelings surrounding thoughts of having a baby are invariably mixed. A "baby" symbolizes both feelings of hope, anticipated maturity, and external verification of internal genital sensations as well as disappointment, inadequacy, and unreality. When a woman finally does become pregnant, the hope of producing a real child is thus inevitably joined with the anxiety that perhaps, as in the past, her baby may turn out not to be a real baby after all.

With the preceding points in mind, it is easy to make the connection between the many novel internal sensations experienced during a first pregnancy and the recurrence of regressive feelings colored by confusion and helplessness. At the same time, the expectant mother's efforts to make sense of these sensations function as a defense against their regressive pull and provide her with a natural impetus for further integration of specifically feminine elements within the personality.

The little girl's initial creation of an imaginary baby as an aid in organizing the confusion or excitement stimulated by her inner genital sensations already reflects an interpersonal structure. The imaginary baby is a personification of internal sense perceptions in human form. Because of this the little girl, just like a real mother, alternately controls and is controlled by her baby (her inner-genital sensations). In this way the interpersonal dynamic appears in relation to the self and the structuring of internal experience as specifically feminine. It leaves the little girl especially prone to orienting her feelings through relationships with someone or something else. Basically, "having a baby"—whether in the imagination, in play, in adolescent activity, or in reality—is intimately bound up with issues of differentiation and integration in feminine identity. From its earliest origins, "having a baby" forms an organizational motif within the personality which is oriented toward interdependence in the sphere of interpersonal relations. The baby relies on the mother for its creation and continued sustenance. The mother relies on her baby for confirmation and integration of her maternal identity. Both the woman's identity as mother and the baby's identity as child develop out of the same matrix of reciprocal interactions over time.

During a first pregnancy this process of reciprocal definition between mother and child is initiated by the fulfillment in reality of earlier wishes or fantasies related to having a child. These earlier imaginings about having a baby can be considered more or less continuous with the actual experience of pregnancy itself. The "baby" lives in its mother's thoughts long before it lives in her womb. From this perspective, discontinuities between the mother's fantasies and the reality of her pregnancy experience can be seen to serve the vital function of supporting her efforts to distinguish between the reality of the child and her internal fantasy of a "baby" at different stages of her own development. The experience of pregnancy thus becomes a period of internal reorientation—a time when the expectant mother's earlier fantasies about having a baby are ideally integrated and brought into alignment with the actual experience of carrying a child inside her.

This internal reorientation shapes the course of pregnancy. It forms the underlying dynamic which ties the events of pregnancy together into the specific pregnancy experience which the expectant mother identifies as her own. Just as earlier fantasies of having a baby provided continuity with the actual experience itself, so the fantasies about the child during pregnancy provide continuity with the newborn infant. Indeed, the subjective experience of women in this study demonstrates that the relationship developed with the fetus during pregnancy is central to the emotional constellation of pregnancy. In this way the development of the woman's sense of her child as a person becomes an end product of her earliest imaginings about having a real baby. Perceiving her child as a person begins the mother's ongoing sense of her child, something which both influences and is influenced by the course of the child's development.

So far this discussion of the integrating force of a first pregnancy has focused on the childhood and adolescent antecedents of pregnancy in feminine intrapsychic experience. But it is equally important to emphasize that neither individual women nor individual mother-child dyads exist apart from their social context or the vicissitudes of their physical experience. Whatever the prospective mother's fantasies about having a baby and however these are used to organize her experience, she has her baby in the context of a particular culture and within the limits of her particular physical constitution. In this sense, a first pregnancy involves the interaction of biological, psychological, and social spheres with each other. These can be thought of as existing in a series of reciprocal feedback systems. Figure 4 shows a diagrammatic representation of reciprocal processes between mother, fetus, and outside world. Naturally, these reciprocal processes occur at all three levels: biological, psychological, and social. The dynamic complexity of this model is difficult to grasp because it attempts to represent a system which, to borrow a phrase coined by Thomas and Chess (1980), is homeodynamic, that is, fluid and changing, oriented toward movement rather than homeostatic balance. This conceptual model views a first pregnancy as a nodal point in a woman's developmental process which cuts across every aspect of her experience. It becomes a dynamic turning point, and from its center the repercussions of having a child radiate out to bring irreversible changes to all levels of her life.

These changes in self-concept and life-style reflect the mores of the contemporary social milieu. Societal structuring of the maternal role in our culture occurs in a framework of values which does little to support or validate the particular vulnerability women feel during pregnancy. The tendency to view pregnancy as an illness or temporary emotional indisposition caused by hormonal shifts ignores the significance a woman her-

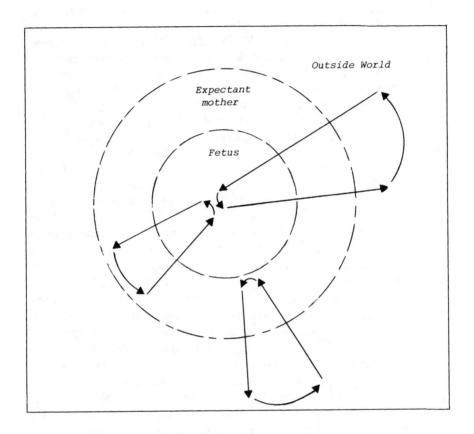

Figure 4   Reciprocal Processes
Between Mother-Fetus and Outside World

Figure 4 depicts the expectant mother, fetus, and environment as
reciprocal feedback systems. Arrows indicate exchange of energy
(stimuli, information) between mother, fetus, and environment
as they function in mutual interaction with one another. Ideally
this figure should be visualized as multidimensional. The interactions shown here are (for the sake of simplicity) drawn with
respect to only one level of experience, but the same reciprocal
feedback systems apply at all levels of experience: biological,
psychological, and social.

self gives to many of her feelings in pregnancy—a significance which, from the results of this study, appear to extend into her relation with the child after childbirth. It also fails to recognize the extent to which pregnancy and the birth of a first child alter the boundaries of a woman's life.

In addition, the negative valuation attached to feelings of dependence, pervasive in our culture which highly values autonomy and individuation, may predispose women to feel more conflict over the amplification of these feelings in pregnancy than might otherwise be the case. The potential value of regressive feelings of dependency is therefore rarely recognized. Such feelings may well serve a progressive outcome. They allow the expectant mother to experience within herself, before her child's birth, feelings of helplessness and vulnerability which replicate the helplessness and vulnerability of her newborn infant. This gives her an experiential base from which to develop an empathic understanding of her infant. Consistent denial or rejection of dependency feelings may render a woman's experience of pregnancy more conflicted or prevent her from getting the support she needs. It may also render the development of empathic attunement to her child's dependency on her more troubled. It is likely that a woman's conflicted response to her own feelings of dependency will reverberate in her response to her baby's dependency on her. Ideally, of course, "good enough" (Winnicott, 1964) mothering involves a variable balance of active and receptive attitudes—the one directed toward the child's needs for structure and nurturance and the other to the child's needs for self-expression and sympathetic understanding.

With reference to these issues, the women in this study are a case in point. Each of them initially struggled to resist her dependency feelings in pregnancy and experienced conflict about finally giving in to what Katherine called her "hedonistic urges" and what Rachael referred to as her "overwhelming passivity." Not one of these women was prepared for the intensity of her dependency feelings as pregnancy progressed, nor did they look upon these feelings as a positive reflection of their developing preoccupation with their unborn child. Although they eventually came to terms with these feelings, they remained inclined to adopt the cultural view that feelings of dependency are basically problematic and somehow "bad." Each woman considered her dependency feelings one of the more difficult aspects of the pregnancy experience to reconcile with her self-esteem. A more accepting attitude toward these feelings might well flow from a conceptual understanding of pregnancy and childbirth as experiences in which mastery and self-esteem on the part of the mother are linked to systematic support from her environment.

Implications for Practice and Research

Theorists concerned with female psychology have defined pregnancy as a period of crisis (Bibring, 1959) or as a developmental phase (Benedek, 1959; Kestenberg, 1975). While these theoretical interpretations are helpful in understanding pregnancy as a time of transition and developmental stress, their focus is primarily oriented toward intrapsychic factors. Concerned with the ways a woman's personality affects her adjustment to pregnancy and the maternal role, they pay less attention to the broad societal factors which contribute to the shaping and structuring of these roles in our society. Sociological literature directed toward understanding the maternal role focuses precisely on these factors but tends to neglect the more psychological aspects of becoming a mother. Given the complexity of the many factors involved, it would seem important to look beyond the limits of individual psychology and the cultural definition of social roles to develop a more comprehensive model of the maternity cycle. Such a model would strike a theoretical balance between psychological explanations aimed at improving or changing mothers and sociological interpretations aimed at making social institutions responsible for the psychological well-being of individuals.

Perhaps such a model as suggested by Leifer (1980) could be similar to that used by ecologists who try to integrate all of the different aspects of any given ecological system by studying the intermodulating factors within the ecology as a whole. It is clear that our present lack of such a theoretical model makes it difficult to accommodate the dynamic interaction of complex variables at different levels of experience which are characteristic of pregnancy as a biopsychological and biosocial event. This makes the typological approach adopted in this study a preliminary to more focused research which can take into account the multiple feedback systems which comprise the pregnant state.

Judging from the experience of women in this study, the symbolic importance of any given pregnancy derives partially from the expectant mother's situation and partially from her view of what this particular pregnancy means to her. Both of these play an important role in her adaptation to pregnancy and the early postpartum period. Findings from this study suggest that psychotherapeutic, obstetrical, and other services directed at pregnant women and new mothers would benefit from deeper understanding of the symbolic importance and developmental significance a woman gives to her pregnancy. Interventions could then be more precisely aimed within this context. Anna, for example, who constellated many of her pregnancy themes around issues of autonomy and individuation in the form of "doing this myself," was supported in her efforts during labor and delivery by the degree of control she felt she had over her environment (largely due to the presence of her physician husband who knew the hospital where she delivered). In contrast, she was traumatized just after delivery by the overly rapid and forceful intervention of a nurse during her first attempts to establish breast-feeding. This prevented her from making this contact in her own way with more respect for her son's own rhythm.

Another practical consideration in formulating interventions made during pregnancy is that of timing. Awareness of the various concerns and vulnerabilities which emerge at different stages of pregnancy as shown in this study would be helpful here. The second trimester, for example, especially the period from 21 to 24 weeks, may be more vulnerable to the development of potential problems in the marital couple than other periods in the pregnancy. Although the second trimester is generally thought of as one of the more satisfying times for woman emotionally, it may in fact also be one of the more subtly difficult periods for the marriage. The increase of internal preoccupation during this time seems linked to increased feelings of distance from men in general and from the husband in particular. Feelings of resentment at having to carry the greater part of the reproductive burden and realization of the limitations on professional aspirations imposed by having a child are more prominent during the second trimester. Greater feelings of dependency starting in the second trimester and continuing throughout the rest of pregnancy and postpartum may also begin to stress the marital balance at this time. Assuming that the middle part of pregnancy is a relatively quiet period because it is physically often an easier time is therefore a mistake.

Findings from this study further suggest that the traditional medical practice of dividing pregnancy into three trimesters, each of three months' duration, does not reflect the emotional dividing lines by which women themselves reckon the experience of pregnancy. With regard to time, two major turning points stand out: The first is the appearance of the fetal movements, and the second is the sudden shift of focus from internal preoccupation with the unborn child to external nesting and preparation for childbirth. This emotionally divides pregnancy into three unequal time segments. Approximately the first four months, or until the first fetal movements are clearly felt, is the "early" part of pregnancy. The next three months constitute the "middle" part of pregnancy, and the last two months with their shift of emotional focus form the "late" part of pregnancy. The striking feature of this emotional, as opposed to medical, division of pregnancy into different time periods is that it closely reflects the mother's emotional experience of her relationship with her unborn child. This supports the view that it is, above all, the developing relation with the fetus which sets the tone of a woman's pregnancy experience and increasingly defines her affective perception of her world.

Recognizing the vitality and emotional significance of this prenatal bond opens up new perspectives on future research. Further exploration of specific continuities between prenatal and postnatal fantasies in women and the characteristics of the babies to which they give birth might begin to demonstrate more direct links between woman's fantasies during pregnancy and their predictive accuracy with regard to their child. All of the women in this study, for example, at one time or another had an accurate fantasy of their child's sex and/or general appearance.

Better understanding of the underlying structural patterns of experience, such as those found in this study (complementarity, initiation, and conflict), would also be helpful. To what extent women individually develop these and to what extent they reflect unconscious structuring mechanisms basic to pregnancy, which are of more evolutionary origin, is uncertain.

In-depth study of what appears as a particularly vulnerable period in pregnancy—approximately between 21 and 24 weeks—is also indicated. It would be interesting to know how prevalent the feelings experienced at this time by women in this study are in a larger population.

Another area for research is the actual importance of having a baby in a woman's life. To date, controversy exists over whether or not a woman can be "fulfilled" without having children. The implied bias of much contemporary psychological thinking favors the view that a woman is somehow incomplete if she does not have a child. More popular traditional female stereotypes also hold this view. The earlier discussion in this chapter about the little girl's fantasy of having a baby as an effort to organize her inner-genital sensations certainly carries with it the implication that only the actual experience of having a baby fully compensates a woman for her disappointment with this fantasy. It further suggests that it is the experience of pregnancy which allows a woman to develop a truly accurate mental representation of her internal reproductive organs and their value. However, the accuracy of this assumption has not been adequately explored. Perhaps the fantasy of having a baby, coupled with real accomplishments in the world, are enough to provide as effective an integrating force in adult female development as the experience of having a real baby.

Conclusion

The problem of the child and its struggle to differentiate physically and psychologically from its mother has been the subject of much research and discussion by modern psychology. The woman's subjective experience of pregnancy and maternity has not received as much attention in spite of its importance and its influence on child-rearing practices.

This study grew out of concern with this problem. Taking the position that motherhood serves to gratify instinctual or biological needs, it also hypothesized that pregnancy presents a woman with developmental issues she seeks to resolve. While infants struggle to differentiate from their mothers in the pursuit of autonomy and individuality, their mothers were likewise seen as struggling to integrate new aspects of themselves generated by entry into the maternal role.

Interviews with women undergoing a first pregnancy provide an opportunity for the direct study of their subjective experiences during this time. Processes which constitute these women's response to pregnancy were identified and the patterns which emerged are seen to be significant for the understanding of pregnancy as an integrating principle in female psychology.

Epilogue

Each of the four women who participated in this study was recontacted between one and two years after this study was conducted. The women were interviewed informally about their experience as mothers and asked what they remembered about their pregnancies.

Predictably, all of them felt more at ease in the maternal role and had established a sense of competence in relation to meeting their child's needs. Still, all of them mentioned that they had never imagined it would take so long to re-establish a sense of their own lives apart from their child. Physically and emotionally they felt it took approximately a year after delivery to really consolidate their maternal identity and regain a feeling of mastery over their bodies and their lives. The one exception to this was Rachael. She felt less hemmed in by her identity as a mother for two reasons: She was already professionally established at the time she became pregnant, and she had an unusually supportive home and work situation. This allowed her to return to work part-time three months after delivery and thus more rapidly resume her interests outside the home. Katherine and Linda were less fortunate. They had difficulty finding early infant child care and so were considerably delayed in their attempts to resume their studies. Each of them mentioned her distress over the situation and emphasized the special difficulties of integrating professional development with maternity. Anna was able to devote herself more fully to the maternal role but felt some anxiety about her continuing lack of professional focus. At the time she was recontacted, she had started her child in a part-time day-care program and was beginning to think about redeveloping some of her earlier interests in music.

Three of the women mentioned that they had started to think about having a second child, although only one of these had actually started planning another pregnancy.

In talking about their memories of their first pregnancy, two women were able to recall many aspects of their experience quite clearly. Of the other two, one woman had some difficulty recalling her early months of pregnancy, but remembered more about the later months when her relationship with the fetus was more developed. The other woman was unable to recall anything other than global impressions of her experience at this time.

What all the women did recall was the feeling of having been diverted from more routine concerns during the period of their pregnancy. They remembered being in touch with a more universal level of experience. In this respect, pregnancy does indeed appear to be a "special" time in a woman's life, a time perhaps marked by uncertainty and difficulty, but also a time of personal transformation and self-discovery.

Appendix A

Proposal for Human Subjects Protection

Submitted to the Committee for Human Subjects Protection

Women participating in this study will be fully informed as to the expected time commitment, regularity of meetings, and the kinds of material collected.

Each woman will be given an extra week after the initial selection interview to reflect on her decision to participate. She will be encouraged to discuss her decision with her husband or others important in her life. Once her decision is made, she will retain the right to decline participation at any time.

The interviewing process has the potential to be a supportive and informative experiment in self-examination. Any of the women who experience psychological stress as a result of the interviewing, or other factors, which are beyond the clinical skills of the researcher will be given appropriate referrals and encouraged to seek more extensive help.

Confidentiality will be assured by deleting all identifying information or labelling from protocols before they are reviewed by independent examiners. Written transcripts of interview material will be made by the researcher and will remain the joint property of the researcher and the respective participant. Women in this study also retain the editorial right to deny disclosure of details they regard as too charged or intimate for presentation.

Potential benefits are felt to outweigh risks. Verny (1981) states that many common emotional stresses seen in normal women during pregnancy are more likely to intensify from not talking enough about their concerns and anxieties than from sharing them in the context of an interested and supportive relationship.

Appendix B

Human Subjects Protection Participation Consent Form

The nature of this research on the effects of a first pregnancy has been fully explained to me. I have been made aware of the expected commitments in time, energy, and personal communication needed for this study. I understand there may be emotional or confidentiality risks involved but feel the benefits of sharing my experience outweigh such risks.

I agree to participate in the weekly, open-ended interviews proposed and understand that written transcripts of these interviews will be made. I give permission to Jellemieke Stauthamer to use this material for her research. I also understand that I may raise questions or decline further participation at any point in the interviewing process and retain the right to deny disclosure of details I consider too personal for presentation.

I understand that the work is being conducted under the auspices of the Wright Institute Graduate School, but that the Wright Institute Graduate School is not liable for any physical injuries directly incurred through my participation in this research. I understand this investigation is in compliance with principles for the protection of human subjects. As such, I understand that all interview material will be handled with respect and strictest confidence.

_____   _____
(Date)   (Participant's Signature)

Appendix C

Notes on the Father's Reaction to the Pregnancy

Some anecdotal references made during this study with respect to the expectant father's experience of his wife's first pregnancy are worthy of mention here.

From the comments made by their wives during the course of their pregnancies about their husbands' reactions to them, it seems that pregnancy affects not only the woman but also her husband in both conscious and unconscious ways. The husband's reactions that were reported seem to fall into two broad categories. One is direct unconscious identification with the wife's condition. The other also derives from processes of identification but is more indirect and symbolic in its manifestation.

A typical example of the first type of reaction manifested by expectant fathers in this study was weight gain. Every one of the subjects' husbands gained significant amounts of weight during his wife's pregnancy—in one case actually going up to 20 pounds over his normal weight. One expectant father also found himself feeling nauseated during the early months of his wife's pregnancy. In addition, three of the women in this study reported that their husbands had had dreams related to the pregnancy.

More indirect or symbolic identification with their wives' condition was also reported. Two of the fathers developed intensely preoccupying hobbies during their wives' pregnancies. One of the other fathers greatly amplified one of his earlier interests in carpentry. During the later months of his wife's pregnancy, he spent many hours tearing their house apart and remodeling it, partly in preparation for the baby and partly just to make improvements. His wife commented wryly on his attitude toward this work. She said she had never seen him be "so intense" about this type of work before. Such intensely preoccupying efforts may mirror the wife's preoccupation with her pregnancy. Tearing out and remodeling the internal structure of the house could also be interpreted as a symbolic enactment of creating something new within, thus replicating the core aspects of the pregnant condition. At the same time, these reactions are defensive in that they allow the husband to experience a sense of purposiveness similar to his wife's.

These comments are anecdotal. They suggest, however, that expectant fathers may experience many aspects of their wives' pregnancy in ways warranting further research. It is unclear to what extent such reactions may predispose a father to involve himself actively with his child once it is born. It also brings out that fathers may be distressed or anxious during their wives' pregnancy in ways requiring defensive strategies. Understanding more about such reactions and their role in preparing the man for fatherhood could be important. Such reactions might demonstrate the extent to which a man's relationship with his child, like the woman's, also begins during pregnancy.

References

Angyal, A. *Neurosis and Treatment: A Holistic Theory.* New York: Wiley & Sons, 1965.

Bachofen, J. [*Myth, Religion and Mother Right*] (R. Manheim, trans.). Princeton, N.J.: Princeton University Press, 1967.

Balinsky, B. I. *An Introduction to Embryology.* Philadelphia, London, Toronto: W. B. Saunders, 1970.

Balint, M. *The Basic Fault: Therapeutic Aspects of Regression.* New York: Brunner/Mazel, 1968.

Balsam, R. H. "Related Issues in Childbearing and Work." *International Journal of Psychoanalytic Psychotherapy* 5 (1976).

Bateson, G. "Some Components of Socialization for Trance." *Ethos* (Sum.) 3: 143–55.

Benedek, T. "Parenthood as a Developmental Phase." *Journal of American Psychoanalytic Association* 7 (1959): 389.

_____ . "The Family as a Psychologic Field." In J. Anthony & T. Benedek, eds., *Parenthood.* Boston: Little, Brown, & Co., 1970.

_____ . "Motherhood and Nurturing." In J. Anthony & T. Benedek, eds., *Parenthood.* Boston: Little, Brown, & Co., 1970.

_____ . "The Psychobiology of Pregnancy." In J. Anthony & T. Benedek eds., *Parenthood.* Boston: Little, Brown, & Co., 1970.

_____ . *Psychosexual Functions in Women.* New York: Ronald Press, 1952.

_____ . "Sexual Functions in Women and Their Disturbance." In S. Arieti, ed., *American Handbook of Psychiatry.* Vol. 1, New York: Basic Books, 1959.

Berelson, B. "Content Analysis." In G. Lindzey, ed., *Handbook of Social Psychology.* Cambridge, Mass.: Addison-Wesley Publishing, 1954.

Berger, P., & Luckmann, T. *The Social Construction of Reality.* Garden City, N.J.: Doubleday, 1966.

Bibring, G. L. "Some Considerations of the Psychological Processes in Pregnancy." In *Psychoanalytic Study of the Child.* Vol. 14. New York: International Universities Press, 1959.

Bibring, G. L.; Dwyer, T. F.; Huntington, D. S.; & Valenstein, F. "A Study of the Psychological Processes in Pregnancy and of the Earliest Mother-Child Relationship." In *Psychoanalytic Study of the Child.* Vol. 14. New York: International Universities Press, 1961.

Bing, E., & Colman, L. *Making Love During Pregnancy.* New York: Bantam Books, 1977.

Blos, P. *On Adolescence: A Psychoanalytic Interpretation.* New York: Free Press, 1962.

Blumer, H. *Symbolic Interactionism: Perspective and Method.* Englewood Cliffs, N.J.: Prentice-Hall, 1969.

Bonaparte, M. *Female Sexuality.* New York: International Universities Press, 1953.

Bonnaud, M., and Reuault D'Allonnes, C. "Vécu Psychologique des Premiers Mouvements de l'Enfant." *Bulletin de la Société Française Psychoprophylaxie Obstetricale* 15 (1963): 43–47.

Bourne, G. *Pregnancy.* London: Cassell & Co., Ltd., 1972.

Bowlby, J. *Attachment and Loss.* London: Hogarth Press, 1969.

Brazelton, B. *Infants and Mothers.* New York: Dell Publishing Co., 1969.

Breen, D. *The Birth of a First Child: Towards an Understanding of Femininity.* London: Tavistock, 1975.

Brewer, G. S., and Brewer, T. *What Every Pregnant Woman Should Know: The Truth About Diets and Drugs in Pregnancy.* New York: Penguin Books, 1979.

Briffault, R. *The Mothers.* New York: Johnson, 1969.

Brody, E. B. "The Meaning of the First Pregnancy for Working-Class Jamaican Women." In W. Miller and L. F. Newman, eds., *The First Child and Family Formation.* North Carolina: University of North Carolina, 1978.

Bronfenbrenner, U. "Toward an Experimental Ecology of Human Development." *American Psychologist* 32 (1977): 519–31.

Brown, J. "Anxiety in Pregnancy." *British Journal of Medical Psychology* 37 (1964): 27–57.

Cameron, P. Age Parameters of Young Adult, Middle-Aged, Old, and Aged. *Journal of Gerontology* 24 (1969): 201–2.

Campbell, D. and Stanley, J. *Experimental and Quasi-Experimental Designs for Research.* Chicago: Rand-McNally, 1963.

Caplan, G. "Emotional Implications of Pregnancy and Influences on Family Relationships." In H. C. Stuart, E. G. Pugh, eds. *The Healthy Child.* Cambridge: Harvard University Press, 1962.

Chapple, P. A., and Furneaux, W. D. "Changes of Personality in Pregnancy and Labour." *Proceedings of the Royal Society of Medicine* 57 (1964): 260–65.

Chassequet-Smirgel, J. *Recherches Psychoanalytiques sur la Sexualité Feminine.* Paris: Payot, 1964.

Chertok, L. *Motherhood and Personality.* London: Tavistock, 1969.

————. "Psychosomatic Aspects of Childbirth." In S. Arieti, ed., *The World Biennial of Psychiatry and Psychotherapy.* Vol. 2. New York: Basic Books, 1973.

Chodorow, N. *The Reproduction of Mothering: Psychoanalysis and the Sociology of Gender.* Berkeley: University of California Press, 1978.

Colman, A., and Colman, L. *Pregnancy: The Psychological Experience.* New York: Seabury Press, 1971.

Colman, L. "Delayed Childbearing: A Descriptive Study of Pregnancy and the Postpartum in Twelve Primiparous Women over Thirty Years Old." Unpublished doctoral dissertation, The Wright Institute, 1978.

Colman, L., and Colman, A. "Pregnancy as an Altered State of Consciousness." *Birth and the Family Journal* 1 (1974): 7.

Cramond, H. "Psychological Aspects of Uterine Dysfunction." *Lancet* 2 (1954): 1241–45.

Davids, A., and Devault, S. "Use of the TAT and Human Figure Drawings in Research on Personality, Pregnancy, and Perception." *Journal of Projective Technique* 4 (1960): 362–65.

————. "Maternal Anxiety During Pregnancy and Childbirth Abnormalities." *Psychosomatic Medicine* 5 (1962): 464–70.

Davids, A.; Devault, S.; and Talmadge, M. "Psychological Study of Emotional Factors in Pregnancy: A Preliminary Report." *Psychosomatic Medicine* 2 (1961): 93–103.

De Beauvoir, S. *The Second Sex.* New York: A. A. Knopf, 1952.

Deutsch, H. *The Psychology of Women.* 2 vols. New York: Grune & Stratton, 1944.

————. *An Introduction to the Discussion of the Psychological Problems of Pregnancy.* New York: Josiam Macy, Jr. Foundation II, 1949.

_____. *Selected Problems of Adolescence*. New York: International Universities Press, 1967.

Dinnerstein, D. *The Mermaid and the Minotaur: Sexual Arrangements and Human Malaise*. New York: Harper & Row, 1976.

Erikson, E. H. "Identity and the Life Cycle: Selected Papers." *Psychological Issues* 1 (1959): 1–171.

_____. *Childhood and Society*, 2nd ed. New York: Norton, 1963.

Fairbairn, W. *The Psychoanalytic Studies of Personality*. London: Tavistock, 1952.

Festinger, L., and Katz, D. eds. *Research Methods in the Behavioral Sciences*. New York: Holt, Rinehart, & Winston, 1953.

Freud, A. *The Ego and the Mechanisms of Defense*. New York: International Universities Press, 1946.

_____. "Normality and Pathology in Childhood: Assessments of Development." In *The Writings of Anna Freud*. Vol. 6. New York: International Universities Press, 1965.

Freud, S. "The Psychology of Women." In *New Introductory Lectures in Psychoanalysis*. New York: Norton, 1933.

_____. The Interpretation of Dreams. In A. A. Brill, ed., *The Basic Writings of Sigmund Freud*. 1900. Reprint. New York: Random House, 1938.

_____. "Totem and Taboo." In A. A. Brill, ed., *The Basic Writings of Sigmund Freud*. 1912. Reprint. New York: Random House, 1938.

_____. "Three Essays on the Theory of Sexuality." In *Standard Edition of the Complete Psychological Works of Sigmund Freud*. Vol. 7. 1905. Reprint. London: Hogarth Press, 1953.

_____. "Some Psychological Consequences of the Anatomical Distinction Between the Sexes." In *Collected papers*. Vol. 5. 1931. Reprint. New York: Basic Books, 1959.

_____. "Female Sexuality." In *Collected papers*. Vol. 5. 1931. Reprint. New York: Basic Books, 1959.

Frey, D. "Being Systematic When You Have But One Subject: Ideographic Method, $N=1$, and All That." *Measurement and Evaluation in Guidance* (April 1973).

Friday, N. *My Mother/My Self: The Daughter's Search for Identity*. New York: Delacorte Press, 1977.

Gillman, R. D. "The Dreams of Pregnant Women and Maternal Adaptation." *American Journal of Orthopsychiatry* 38: (1968) 688–92.

Giorgi, A.; Fischer, C.; and Murray, E. eds. *Duquesne Studies in Phenomenological Psychology*, Vol. 2. Pittsburgh: Duquesne University Press, 1975.

Glaser, B., and Strauss, A. *The Discovery of Grounded Theory*. Chicago: Aldine Publishing Co., 1967.

Glick, P. C. "A Demographer Looks at American Families." *Journal of Marriage and the Family* 2 (1975): 37/1.

_____. "Updating of Life Cycle of the Family. *Journal of Marriage and the Family* 2 (1977): 39/1.

Gordon, R. E. "Factors in Postpartum Emotional Adjustment." *American Journal of Orthopsychiatry* 37 (1967): 359–60.

Gordon, R. E., and Gordon, K. K. "Social Factors in the Prediction and Treatment of Emotional Disorders of Pregnancy." *American Journal of Obstetrics and Gynaecology* 77 (1959): 1074–83.

Green, R. T. "Perceived Styles of Mother-Daughter Relationship and the Prenatal Adjustment of the Primigravida." Unpublished doctoral dissertation, George Washington University, 1973.

Greenacre, P. *Trauma, Growth, and Personality*. New York: Norton, 1952.

Gressot, M. "Aspects Psychologiques de l'ASD." *Bulletin de la Société Internationale Psychoprophylaxie Obstetricale* 1 (1959): 43–75.

Grimm, E. "Psychologic and Social Factors in Pregnancy, Delivery and Outcome." In S. Richardson and A. Guttmacher, *Childbearing—Its Social and Psychological Aspects.* Baltimore: Williams & Wilkins, 1967.

Grof, S. "Prenatal Memory." In *Realms of the Human Unconscious.* New York: E. P. Dutton, 1976.

Groffman, K. "Life-Span Development Psychology in Europe: Past and Present. "In L. R. Goulet and P. B. Baltes eds., *Life-Span Developmental Psychology: Research and Theory.* New York: Academic Press, 1970.

Gould, R. *Transformations: Growth and Change in Adult Life.* New York: Simon & Schuster, 1978.

Guntrip, H. *Psychoanalytic Theory, Therapy, and the Self.* London: Hogarth Press, 1971.

Hamilton, M. "The Late Baby Boom." *San Francisco Sunday Examiner and Chronicle,* July 12, 1981, section A: 1–4.

Hanford, J. M. "Pregnancy as a State of Conflict." *Psychological Reports* 22 (1968): 1313–42.

Hansen, N. *Patterns of Discovery.* Cambridge: Harvard University Press, 1958.

Harding, E. *Woman's Mysteries: Ancient and Modern.* New York: Harper & Row, 1971.

Harlow, H. F. "Affectional Responses in the Infant Monkey." *Science* 130 (1959): 421.

Horney, K. *Feminine Psychology* (Harold Kelman, ed.). New York: Norton, 1967.

Howells, J. C., ed. *Modern Perspectives in Psycho-Obstetrics.* New York: Brunner/Mazel, 1972.

Jarrahi-Zadek, A.; Kane, F.; Van de Castle, R.; La ChenBruch, P.; and Ewing, J. "Emotional and Cognitive Changes in Pregnancy and Early Puerperium." *British Journal of Psychiatry* 115 (1969): 797–805.

Jeffcoate, J. In Sir E. L. Holland and A. W. Bourne eds., *British Obstetric and Gynaecological Practice,* 2 vols. Vol. 1, *Obstetrics.* London: Heinemann, 1963.

Jessner, L.; Weigert, E.; and Foy, J. "The Development of Parental Attitudes During Pregnancy." In J. Anthony and T. Benedek, eds., *Parenthood.* Boston: Little, Brown, & Co., 1970.

Joffe, J. M. *Prenatal Determinants of Behavior.* Oxford: Pergamon Press, 1969.

Jones, E. "Early Development of Female Sexuality." In *Papers on Psychoanalysis.* London: Balliere Tindall & Cox, 1938.

Jung, C. G. "The Stages of Life." In J. Campbell, ed., *The Portable Jung.* 1933. Reprint. New York: Viking Press, 1971.

—————. Dreams (R. F. C. Hull, trans.). In *The Collected works of C. G. Jung.* Vols. 4, 8, 12, 16). Bollingen Series no. 20. 1916-1945. Reprint. Princeton, N.J.: Princeton University Press, 1974.

Jung, C. G., and Kerenyi, C. *Essays on a Science of Mythology* (R. F. C. Hull, trans.). 1949. Reprint. Princeton, N.J.: Princeton University Press, 1969.

Kammerer, T. "La Psychologie de la Douleur." *Bulletin de la Société Française Psychoprophylaxie Obstetricale* 15 (1963): 115–22.

Kaplan, L. *Oneness and Separateness: From Infant to Individual.* New York: Simon & Schuster, 1978.

Kear-Colwell, J. J. "Neuroticism in the Early Puerperium." *British Journal of Psychiatry* 3 (1965): 1189–92.

Kelly, G. A. *The Psychology of Personal Constructs.* New York: Norton, 1955.

Kestenberg, J. S. *Children and Parents: Psychoanalytic Studies in Development.* New York: Jason Aronson, 1975.

Klein, H.; Potter, H.; and Dyk, R. *Anxiety in Pregnancy and Childbirth*. New York: Hoeber, 1952.

Klein, M., and Riviere, J. *Love, Hate and Reparation*. London: Hogarth, 1937.

Kogan, W. S.; Boe, E. E.; and Gocka, E. F. "Personality Changes in Unwed Mothers Following Parturition." *Journal of Clinical Psychology* 1 (1968): 2–11.

Kogan, W. S.; Boe, E. E.; and Valentine, B. L. "Changes in the Self-Concept of Unwed Mothers." *Journal of Psychology* 59 (1965): 3–10.

Kramer, M., et al. "Do Dreams Have Meaning? An Empirical Study." *American Journal of Psychiatry* (July 1976) 778–81.

Kubie, L. *Psychoanalysis as Science*. New York: Basic Books, 1952.

Lazarre, J. *The Mother Knot*. New York: McGraw-Hill, 1976.

Leboyer, F. *Birth Without Violence*. New York: Alfred A. Knopf, 1976.

Leifer, M. *Psychological Effects of Motherhood: A Study of First Pregnancy*. New York: Praeger Publishers, 1980.

Levinson, D. J. The Mid-life Transition: A Period in Adult Psychosocial Development. *Psychiatry* 40 (1977): 99–112.

Levinson, D. J., et al. *The Seasons of a Man's Life*. New York: Alfred A. Knopf, 1978.

Lewin, K. *Field Theory in Social Science*. (D. Cartwright, ed.). New York: Harper & Row, 1951.

Lewis, A. *An Interesting Condition*. New York: Doubleday, 1950.

Lifton, R. *The Life of the Self: Toward a New Psychology*. New York: Simon & Schuster, 1976.

Lindgren, H. C. "Measuring Need to Achieve by N ACH-N AFF Scale–A Forced-choice Questionnaire." *Psychological Reports* 39 (1976): 907–10.

Loesch, J. G., and Greenberg, N. H. "Areas of Conflict Observed during Pregnancy." *American Journal of Orthopsychiatry* 32 (1962): 624–36.

Lomas, P. The Husband-Wife Relationship in Cases of Puerperal Breakdown. *British Journal of Medical Psychology* 32 (1959): 117–23.

_____. "The Concept of Maternal Love." *Psychiatry* 3 (1962): 256–62.

_____. "The Significance of Post-Partum Breakdown." In *The Predicament of the Family*. London: Hogarth Press, 1972.

Lukesch, M. "Psychologic Faktoren der Schwangerschaft." Unpublished doctoral dissertation, University of Salzburg, 1975.

McCall, R. *Infants. The New Knowledge*. Cambridge: Harvard University Press, 1979.

McCauley, C. S. *Pregnancy After 35*. New York: Dutton, 1976.

McConnell, O. L., and Daston, P. "Body Image Changes in Pregnancy." *Journal of Projective Technique* 25 (1961): 451–56.

McDonald, R.L. "The Role of Emotional Factors in Obstetric Complications: A Review." *Psychosomatic Medicine* 20 (1968): 222–237.

McGoldrick, M. "The Joining of Families Through Marriage: The New Couple." In E. Carter & M. McGoldrick eds., *The Family Life Cycle*. New York: Gardner Press, 1980.

Macfarlane, A. "The Psychology of Childbirth." In J. Bruner, M. Cole, & B. Lloyd eds., *The Developing Child*. Cambridge: Harvard University Press, 1977.

Mahler, M. S. "Thoughts About Development and Individuation." *Psychoanalytic study of the Child* 18 (1963): 307–24.

_____. *On Human Symbiosis and the Vicissitudes of Individuation*. New York: International Universities Press, 1968.

Malinowski, B. *The Sexual Life of Savages*. New York: Harcourt, Brace & World, 1929.

Mead, G. H. *George Herbert Mead on Social Psychology: Selected Papers* (A. Strauss, ed.) Chicago: University of Chicago Press, 1964. (Originally published 1934.)

Mead, M. *Male and Female.* London: Victor Gollancz, 1949.

Mead, M. and Newton, N. "Conception, Pregnancy, Labour and the Puerperium in Cultural Perspective." In *Médecine Psychosomatique et Maternité* (Proceedings of the First International Congress of Psychosomatic Medicine and Childbirth, Paris, July 8–12, 1962). Paris: Gauthier-Villars, 1965.

Mann, E. C. "Psychiatric Investigation of Habitual Abortion." *Obstetrics and Gynecology* 7 (1956): 589.

Menninger, W. C. The Emotional Factors in Pregnancy. *Menninger Clinic Bulletin* 7 (1943): 15–24.

Miller, R. "The Eye-Blink Reflex of the Rat in the Hydroid Campanularia." *Journal of Experimental Zoology* 162 (1969): 23–44.

Miller, W. B., and Newman, L. F. eds. *The First Child and Family Formation.* North Carolina: University of North Carolina, 1978.

Montagu, A. *Touching: The Human Significance of Skin.* New York: Columbia University Press, 1971.

Morgan, P. E. "The Relationship of the Primipara to Her Mother: A Case Study Approach." Unpublished doctoral dissertation. California School of Professional Psychology, Berkeley, 1979.

Neumann, E. *The Great Mother.* 1955. Reprint. Princeton, N.J.: Princeton University Press, 1972.

Newman, L. F. "Symbolism and Status Change: Fertility and the First Child in India and the United States." In W. Miller and L. F. Newman eds., *The First Child and Family Formation.* North Carolina: University of North Carolina, 1978.

Newton, N. *Maternal Emotions.* New York: Hoeber, 1955.

————. "Interrelationships Between Sexual Responsiveness, Birth and Breast Feeding." In J. Zubin and J. Money, *Contemporary Sexual Behavior: Critical Issues in the '70's.* Baltimore: Johns Hopkins University Press, 1973.

Pavenstedt, E. Progress Report. USPHS grant application. March 1959 (unpublished).

————. The Effect of Maternal Maturity and Immaturity on Child Development. USPHS grant application. September 1959-August 1964 (unpublished).

Perlman, H. H. *Personal Social Role and Personality.* Chicago: University of Chicago Press, 1968.

Piaget, J. *The Construction of Reality in the Child.* New York: Basic Books, 1959.

Pines, D. "The Relevance of Early Psychic Development to Pregnancy and Abortion." *International Journal of Psycho-Analysis* 63 (1982): 311–19.

Racamier, P. C. A Propos de Maternité et Sexe de Marie Langer. *Evolution Psychiatrique* 1 (1953): 559–65.

————. "Troubles de la Sexualité Feminine et du Sens Maternel." *Bulletin de la Société Française de Psychoprophylaxie Obstetricale* 432 (1967): 1–40.

Ralph, N. "The Clinical Method: A Naturalistic Phenomenological Technique for Psychology." Doctoral dissertation, The Wright Institute, 1976. *Dissertation Abstracts International* 37 (1977): 5371B (University Microfilms No. 77-6548).

Rank, O. *The Trauma of Birth.* London: Kegan Paul, 1939.

Rapaport, D. "Perception of Pain and Some Factors that Modify It." In H. Abramson ed., *Problems of Consciousness.* New York: Josiah Macy Foundation, 1951.

Read, G. D. *Natural Childbirth.* London: Heinemann, 1933.

Rich, A. *Of Woman Born: Motherhood as Experience and Institution.* New York: W. W. Norton, 1976.

Ringrose, C. "Psychosomatic Influence in the Genesis of Toxaemia of Pregnancy." *Canadian Medical Association Journal* 84: (1961).

Rosenblatt, J., and Lehrman, D. S. "Mother-Young Synchrony in Rats." In H. Rheingold ed., *Maternal Behavior in Mammals*. New York: John Wiley, 1963.

Rossi, A. S. "Transition to Parenthood." *Journal of Nursing* 70 (1970): 506.

Rottman, G. "Untersuchungen über Einstellung zur Schwangerschaft und zur Fotalen Entwiklung." In H. Graber ed., *Geist und Psyche*. Munich: Kindler Verlag, 1974.

Rubin, L. *Women of a Certain Age*. New York: Harper & Row, 1979.

Rubin, R. "Attainment of the Maternal Role, Processes, Models and Referrants." *Nursing Research* 16 (1967): 237–45, 342–46.

Salk, L. "The Effects of the Normal Heartbeat Sound on the Behavior of the Newborn Infant: Implications for Mental Health." *World Mental Health* 12 (1960): 168.

Scully, D., and Bart, P. "A Funny Thing Happened on the Way to the Orifice: Women in Gynecology Textbooks." *American Journal of Sociology* 78 (1973): 1045–50.

Sechehaye, M. A. *Symbolic Realization*. New York: International Universities Press, 1951.

Serkin, E. "Personality Development in Highly Educated Women in the Years Eighteen to Forty-Five." Unpublished doctoral dissertation, The Wright Institute, 1980.

Shainess, N. "Psychological Problems Associated with Motherhood." In S. Arieti et al., eds., *American Handbook of Psychiatry*. Vol. 3. New York: Basic Books, 1966.

Shainess, N. "Women's Liberation—and Liberated Woman." In S. Arieti, ed., *The World Biennial of Psychiatry and Psychotherapy*. Vol. 2. New York: Basic Books, 1973.

Shatzman, L., and Strauss, A. *Field Research: Strategies for a Natural Society*. Englewood Cliffs, N.J.: Prentice-Hall, 1973.

Sheehy, G. *Passages: Predictable Crises of Adult Life*. New York: Bantam Books, 1976.

Shereshefski, P., and Yarrow, L. J. *Psychological Aspects of a First Pregnancy and Early Postnatal Adaptation*. New York: Raven Press, 1973.

Sherman, J. A. *On the Psychology of Women: A Survey of Empirical Studies*. Springfield, Ill.: Charles C. Thomas, 1971.

Sontag, L. W. "Significance of Foetal Environmental Differences. *American Journal of Obstetrics and Gynaecology* 42 (1941): 996–1003.

_____. "War and the Fetal Maternal Relationship." *Marriage and Family Living* 6 (1944): 1–5.

_____. "Implications of Fetal Behavior and Environment for Adult Personalities." *Annals of New York Academy of Sciences* (February 1966): 782–86.

Spiegelberg, H. *Phenomenology in Psychology and Psychiatry*. Evanston, Ill.: Northwestern University Press, 1972.

Sullivan, H. S. *The Interpersonal Theory of Psychiatry*. New York: Norton, 1953.

Telgenhof, G. "De Godin der Huishouding in de 19de Eeuw." *NRC Handelsblad* (24 Oct. 1981).

Thomas, A., and Chess, S. *The Dynamics of Psychological Development*. New York: Brunner/Mazel, 1980.

Thomas, H. *Training for Childbirth: A Program of Natural Childbirth with Rooming-in*. New York: McGraw-Hill, 1950.

Treadway, C. R.; Kane, F. J.; Jarrahi-Zadeh, A.; Jarrahi-Zadeh, L.; and Morris, A." A Psychoendocrine Study of Pregnancy and the Puerperium." *American Journal of Psychiatry* 125 (1969): 480–86.

Trethowan, W. H., and Dickens, C. "Cravings, Aversions, and Pica of Pregnancy." in J. Howells, ed., *Modern Perspectives in Psycho-Obstetrics*. New York: Brunner/Mazel, 1972.

Vaillant, G. *Adaptation to Life*. Boston: Little, Brown, 1978.

Verny, T. *The Secret Life of the Unborn Child*. New York: Summit Books, 1981.

Vygotsky, L. S. *Mind in Society*. Cambridge: Harvard University Press, 1978.

Watson, A. "A Psychiatric Study of Idiopathic Prolonged Labour." *Obstetrics and Gynaecology* 13 (1959): 589–95.

Weiss, R. S. "Issues in Holistic Research." In H. S. Becker, ed., *Institutions and the Person: Papers Presented to Everett C. Hughes*. Chicago: Aldine, 1968.

West, U., ed. *Women in a Changing World*. New York: McGraw-Hill, 1975.

White, B. *The First Three Years of Life*. Englewood Cliffs, N.J.: Prentice-Hall, 1975.

Winnicott, D. W. "Primary Maternal Preoccupation." In *Collected Papers: Through Paediatrics to Psycho-Analysis*. London: Tavistock, 1958.

―――――. *The Child, the Family and the Outside World*. New York: Pelican, 1964.

―――――. *The Maturational Processes and the Facilitating Environment: Studies in the Theory of Emotional Development*. London: Hogarth, 1965.

―――――. "The Mother-Infant Experience of Mutuality." In J. Anthony and T. Benedek, eds., *Parenthood*. Boston: Little, Brown, 1970.

Worell, L., and Worell, J. "The Parent Behavior Form". Unpublished manual, University of Kentucky, 1974.

Zemlick, M. J., and Watson, R. "Maternal Attitudes of Acceptance and Rejection During and After Pregnancy". *American Journal of Orthopsychiatry* 23 (1953): 570.

Zilboorg, G. Depressive Reactions Related to Parenthood. *Research in Nervous and Mental Disorders* 11 (1931): 413–49.

Index